Obst and Gynaecology

Cas tions and C ntaries

Obstetrics and Gynaecology

Cases, Questions and Commentaries

Philip N. Baker B MedSci, BMBS, MRCOG, DM
Professor/Honorary Consultant Obstetrician and Gynaecologist
Department of Obstetrics and Gynaecology
City Hospital
Nottingham, UK

Toby N. Fay MBBS, MD, MRCOG
Consultant Obstetrician and Gynaecologist
Department of Obstetrics and Gynaecology
City Hospital
Nottingham, UK

Robert H. Hammond FRCS (Ed), MRCOG
Consultant Obstetrician and Gynaecologist
Department of Obstetrics and Gynaecology
University Hospital
Nottingham, UK

WB Saunders Company Limited
Edinburgh   London   New York   Philadelphia   St Louis   Sydney   Toronto

WB SAUNDERS
An imprint of Harcourt Publishers Limited

© 1998 WB Saunders Company Limited
© 1999 Harcourt Publishers Limited

First published 1998
Reprinted 1999

ISBN 0702 02235 7

British Library Cataloguing in Publication Data
A catalogue record for this book is available from the British Library

Library of Congress Cataloging in Publication Data
A catalog record for this book is available from the Library of Congress

Printed in Great Britain by WBC Book Manufacturers, Bridgend,
Mid-Glamorgan

Contents

Section 3: Gynaecological problems   149

Foreword

How do doctors learn to manage their patients' problems effectively? Traditionally universities have expected medical students to assimilate large volumes of knowledge encompassing basic sciences, detailed pathology, as well as the theoretical basis of medicine and surgery. Students and young doctors have been expected to apply their knowledge to practical clinical problems, learning mainly by apprenticeship; observing and copying, rather than being formally trained. Undergraduate and postgraduate examinations concentrate on knowledge (sometimes obscure) and assessment of clinical skills, usually learnt by rote and displayed in an artificial situation. True understanding is rarely tested effectively.

However, times are changing. New curricula are springing up which reflect an emphasis on problem-based learning, interactive teaching methods and understanding. Postgraduates preparing for professional examinations such as the MRCOG part II examinations now find themselves asked to justify or critically appraise rather than merely discuss. Many candidates find difficulty with this because of the type of training that they have received in the past. Although "what" is still an important question "why" is at least its equal.

The clinical cases presented in *Obstetrics and Gynaecology: Cases, Questions and Commentaries* lead the trainee into a series of questions which allow the reader to interact with the problem, seeing if they know what to do and why. After any form of question and answer, readers are anxious to see whether they were correct and are led into the commentary which is designed not just to present the answers to the original questions but also to provide the background knowledge to put the case in context with basic sciences and other clinical information. Knowledge is thus presented in context. The relevance is immediately apparent and is all the more memorable for it. By working through the typical clinical cases presented in this book, trainees will develop a solid understanding of obstetrics and gynaecology and should be able to manage their patients more effectively.

I. R. Johnson
Nottingham

Preface

The idea for this book evolved from a discussion between the authors regarding the changes in the training structure in obstetrics and gynaecology. We all expressed concern that these changes may lead to reduced clinical exposure and, ultimately, to a reduction in clinical experience. With this in mind, we set about producing a set of fifty cases from which we have raised questions for trainees and candidates to assess. These are all cases in which the authors have been involved with over the last few years. In addition to facilitating a greater exposure to clinical cases of obstetrics and gynaecology, we also hope that the book will help candidates pass postgraduate examinations. The latter aim is particularly pertinent in view of the changes to the membership examination of the Royal College of Obstetricians and Gynaecologists.

Ideally, we suggest that readers work through each case with pencil and paper. We think maximum benefit will be achieved if readers commit themselves on paper to the questions raised in the case histories, before going on to the commentaries and subsequent answers. A limited number of references have been provided; some of these are useful review articles, some are important papers, often of historical interest, which have altered clinical practice.

Philip N Baker
Toby N Fay
Robert H Hammond

List of abbreviations

AC	abdominal circumference
ACTH	adrenocorticotrophic hormone
AITP	autoimmune thrombocytopenic purpura
ANA	antinuclear antibody
APA	antiplatelet antibody
APL	acute promyelocytic leukaemia
APTT	activated partial thromboplastin time
ATRA	all-trans retinoic acid
BPD	biparietal diameter
BMI	body mass index
bpm	beats per minute
CIN	cervical intraepithelial neoplasia
CMV	cytomegalovirus
CT	computed tomography
CTG	cardiotocograph
CVP	central venous pressure
CVS	chorionic villus sampling
DHEAS	dihydroepiandrostenedione sulphate
DIC	disseminated intravascular coagulation
DNA	deoxyribonucleic acid
DUB	dysfunctional uterine bleeding
EPI	echo-planar imaging
FL	femur length
FSH	follicle stimulating hormone
HC	head circumference
hCG	human chronic gonadotrophin
HELLP	haemolysis, elevated liver enzymes and low platelet count (syndrome)
HIV	human immunodeficiency virus
HMG	human menopausal gonadotrophin
ICP	intrahepatic cholestasis of pregnancy
ICSI	intracytoplasmic sperm injection
Ig	immunoglobulin
INR	international normalized ratio
IQ	intelligence quotient

ITP	idiopathic thrombocytopenic purpura
IUCD	intrauterine contraceptive device
IUD	intrauterine device
IUGR	intrauterine growth restriction
IVF	*in vitro* fertilization
IVP	intravenous pyelogram
KCT	kaolin clotting time
LH	luteinizing hormone
LHRH	luteinizing hormone releasing hormone
LLETZ	large loop excision of the transformation zone
LOAH	late-onset adrenal hyperplasia
MCH	mean corpuscular haemoglobin
MCV	mean corpuscular volume
MRI	magnetic resonance imaging
17-OHP	17-hydroxyprogesterone
PAIgG	platelet-associated IgG
PCV	packed cell volume
Po_2	partial pressure of oxygen
PPET	prophylactic partial exchange transfusion
RCOG	Royal College of Obstetricians and Gynaecologists
SaO_2	arterial haemoglobin oxygen saturation
SGA	small for gestational age
SHGB	sex hormone binding globulin
SLE	systemic lupus erythematosus
TNF	tumour necrosis factor
TORCH	toxoplasmosis, rubella, cytomegalovirus, herpes (screen)
TPO-Ab	thyroid peroxidase antibody
TSH	thyroid stimulating hormone
TTP	thrombotic thrombocytopenic purpura
VAIN	vaginal intraepithelial neoplasia
VDRL	Venereal Disease Reference Laboratory
VIN	vulval intraepithelial neoplasia
VZIG	varicella zoster immune globulin

SECTION I

▶ **Problems in pregnancy**

CASE I

Prenatal diagnostic testing

A 25-year-old P1 + 1 woman attended the postnatal clinic 6 weeks after a normal delivery. Her first pregnancy had ended in a spontaneous miscarriage at 10 weeks' gestation. Her second pregnancy resulted in the delivery of a child with Down's syndrome who died shortly after birth from complications of a congenital heart defect. The puerperium had been otherwise uncomplicated. She and her husband were concerned about the likelihood of a recurrence in any future pregnancy.

QI: What is the risk of Down's syndrome in any future pregnancy likely to be?

Q2:   Which of the following statements regarding Down's syndrome are correct?
A: The majority of individuals have an IQ of less than 50 at 10 years of age.
B: The incidence of Alzheimer's disease is increased.
C: The incidence of congenital heart defects is about 40%.
D: The incidence of acute leukaemia is increased.
E: The ratio of females:males is above that of the general population.
F: The finding of a horseshoe kidney is characteristic.

Q3:   How would you evaluate this couple to establish their risk of having a chromosomally abnormal child?

A chromosomal study had been performed on the child, and had found that the extra chromosome 21 material was not present as a separate chromosome but as a translocation on chromosome 14. Cytogenetic studies of the couple revealed that the father carried a balanced translocation between chromosomes 14 and 21.

Q4:   Which of the following statements regarding the risk of Down's syndrome in any future pregnancy are correct?
A: The theoretical risk of a child with Down's syndrome is 25%.
B: The actual risk of a child with Down's syndrome is lower than the theoretical risk.
C: The risk is lower than if the mother carried the translocation.
D: The risk is not influenced by maternal age.
E: If the translocation had been between the two 21 chromosomes, the theoretical risk would be 50%.

Nine months later, the patient attended the antenatal booking clinic (at 8 weeks' gestation) with her husband.

Q5: What prenatal diagnostic procedure would you advise?

Q6: Which of the following statements regarding early amniocentesis (before 15 weeks' gestation) are correct?
A: The sampling failure rate is approximately 5%.
B: The culture failure rate is approximately 5%.
C: Contamination by maternal cells is less likely than if chorionic villus sampling is used.
D: The proportion of viable fetal cells is dependent on the gestational age at sampling.

Q7: Which of the following statements regarding chorionic villus sampling are correct?
A: To assess fetal karyotype, 50–100 mg of chorionic villi is needed.
B: There is a 5% incidence of placental mosaicism.
C: Cytogenetic results can be obtained after 24 hours.
D: Trophoblast cells have a higher mitotic rate than amniocytes.

After considering the different options, the couple opted for chorionic villus sampling, which was performed at 11 weeks' gestation. The transabdominal procedure was uncomplicated, and the fetal karyotype was subsequently reported as 46XX.

Q8: Which of the following complications is the pregnancy at an increased risk of (relative to the general pregnant population)?
A: Severe fetal limb abnormalities.
B: Miscarriage.
C: Neonatal pulmonary complications.
D: Orthopaedic deformities of the newborn.

A detailed ultrasound scan at 18 weeks' gestation was unremarkable, and the patient's subsequent antenatal course was uncomplicated. After a spontaneous labour, a female infant weighing 3.45 kg was delivered normally at 40 weeks' gestation.

COMMENTARY

Down's syndrome has an prevalence of about 1 in 700 live births. In 95% of cases, it is the result of trisomy 21, with the extra chromosome being of paternal origin in 20–25% of cases. In women aged 25 years, the overall risk of a child born with Down's syndrome is approximately 1:1350, and the risk of a Down's syndrome fetus at mid-trimester is approximately 1:1080. The risk of Down's syndrome, as well as other chromosomal abnormalities, increases significantly with advancing maternal age. However, once a couple has had a child with Down's syndrome, the risk that subsequent progeny will have a chromosomal abnormality (trisomy 21 or other) is in the range of 1%, assuming the parental chromosomal complements are normal (**Q1**).

Down's syndrome is the most common congenital cause of intellectual impairment; although there is some individual variation, in most cases the IQ is less than 50 at 10 years of age. Moreover, there is increasing evidence that the incidence of Alzheimer's disease in Down's syndrome is high. In addition to the learning disability, structural anomalies may be present; those involving the heart occur in 40%. The frequency of acute leukaemia amongst individuals with Down's syndrome is higher than that in the general population. The majority of cases are of the lymphoblastic type. A preponderance of females is found in trisomy 18, not trisomy 21. Similarly, horseshoe kidneys are characteristically found in Edwards' syndrome rather than Down's syndrome (**Q2: true = B, C, D; false = A, E, F**).

The evaluation of a couple who have had a child born with Down's syndrome is often performed in conjunction with a clinical geneticist. It is particularly important to determine whether the chromosomal complement of the child was established. If the child were found to have a translocation, then the 1% risk applicable to cases of trisomy 21 would not be relevant. If chromosomal analysis of the child is not available, the couple should undergo cytogenetic studies to determine whether either of them is a balanced carrier of a structural chromosomal rearrangement. You should take a careful family history. This includes enquiries about the health status of the couple and their relatives. You should exclude any consanguinity in the family. You may need to obtain medical records to confirm the nature of any medical disorder in family members (**Q3**).

Translocations are found in about 5% of individuals with Down's syndrome; there is no evidence of phenotypic differences between trisomic and translocation cases of Down's syndrome. Maternal age is not a factor in such cases as non-dysjunction is not the cause. Among cases of Down's syndrome due to translocation, about half arise *de novo*, and about half are inherited from a balanced translocation carrier parent. If inherited, the recurrence risk depends on the chromosomes involved and which parent is the carrier. Theoretically, if a parent has a translocation between chromosomes 14 and 21, 25% of fetuses will be normal, 25% will be carriers, 25% will have Down's syndrome and 25% will have no chromosome 21 material. However, absence of chromosome 21 material is not compatible with life; thus the theoretical risk of a child with Down's syndrome is 33%. The empirical risk is considerably lower. If the father carries the translocation, the risk is 2%. If the mother had been the carrier, the risk would have been 10% (Boue and Gallano, 1984). The deviation from the theoretical risk probably results from an increased chance of a Down's fetus aborting spontaneously (which may have been the case in her first pregnancy). The explanation for the lower risk when the father is the carrier is unclear. If either parent carries a translocation between the two chromosomes 21, the risk of either a child with Down's syndrome or a spontaneous miscarriage is virtually 100% (**Q4: true = B, C, D; false = A, E**).

You should not advise the couple to have any particular diagnostic procedure! Your job is to provide accurate information and non-directive counselling as to the different options that are available (**Q5**).

Traditionally, amniocentesis has been performed between 15 and 17 weeks' gestation, when the fundus is readily accessible abdominally, and abnormal results are known before 20 weeks' gestation. Recognition of some of the disadvantages of chorionic villus biopsy has led to interest in early amniocentesis (before 15 weeks' gestation). Using ultrasonographic guidance, early amniocentesis is technically easy; the failure rate in sampling amniotic fluid has been consistently estimated to be below 2%. Some operators use 22-gauge needles to avoid stripping the membrane from the uterus, aspirate slowly to prevent the amniotic sac collapsing, and remove fluid volumes of only 1 ml per week of gestation. Between 11 and 14 weeks' gestation, the cytogenetic failure rate has been reported to be as low as 0.3% (Johnson and Godmilow, 1988), although at earlier gestations the failure rate is higher. Although fewer cells are obtained at earlier gestations, the proportion of viable cells does not change significantly with gestation between 8 and 18 weeks. Early amniocentesis is associated with lower rates of maternal contamination and pseudomosaicism than chorionic villus sampling. Fetal loss rates do not seem to be significantly higher than if the procedure is performed after 15 weeks' gestation, but concerns relating to possible increased rates of neonatal pulmonary complications and orthopaedic deformities have been raised (**Q6: true = C; false = A, B, D**).

Chorion frondosum or placental tissue is an alternative to amniotic fluid for prenatal diagnosis of genetic disorders. The transabdominal route is now the most popular. To assess fetal karyotype, 5–10 mg of chorionic villi are needed. Chorionic villus sampling enables rapid cytogenetic analysis due to the higher mitotic activity of trophoblast cells compared with amniocytes. Cytogenetic results are obtained from spontaneous mitoses in direct preparations, or after short-term culture for 12–24 hours. Long-term culture (up to 7 days) ensures specimens of sufficient quality for banding studies, but is complicated by maternal contamination in up to 10% of cases. There is a 1–2% incidence of confined placental or pseudomosaicism, where a discrepancy exists between chorionic and fetal karyotypes, necessitating further investigation by amniocentesis. In most cases, an aneuploid or polyploid mosaic is identified in the chorion, whereas the fetal karyotype is normal (**Q7: true = C, D; false = A, B**).

Randomized and controlled trials suggest that the fetal loss rate after chorionic villus sampling is slightly higher than that after amniocentesis. As would be anticipated, this discrepancy is lowest in centres where operators have the greatest experience. The procedure-related loss rate over women who do not have chorionic villus sampling is between 1 and 2%. An additional concern about the safety of chorionic villus sampling was raised by the report of severe limb abnormalities in babies whose mothers had undergone early (less than 66 days' gestation) transabdominal sampling (Firth et al., 1991). Different subsequent reports have confirmed or dismissed this initial observation, but there is no evidence to suggest that these complications occur when the procedure is performed at 11 weeks' gestation. As discussed above, neonatal pulmonary complications and orthopaedic deformities of the newborn are suggested complications of early amniocentesis (**Q8: true = B; false = A, C, D**).

REFERENCES

Boue A, Gallano P. A collaborative study of the segregation of inherited chromosome structural rearrangements in 13 356 prenatal diagnoses. *Prenat Diagn* 1984; **4**: 45–67.

Firth HV, Boyd PA, Chamberlain P, MacKenzie IZ, Lindembaum RH, Huson SM. Severe limb abnormalities after chorion villus sampling at 56–66 days' gestation. *Lancet* 1991; **337**: 762–763.

Johnson A, Godmilow L. Genetic amniocentesis at 14 weeks or less. *Clin Obstet Gynecol* 1988; **31**: 345–352.

FACTS YOU SHOULD HAVE LEARNT . . .

▶ How to evaluate a couple to establish their risk of a second chromosomally abnormal child
▶ The risks of Down's syndrome in different clinical situations
▶ The complications of Down's syndrome
▶ The advantages and disadvantages of early amniocentesis
▶ The advantages and disadvantages of chorionic villus sampling

CASE 2

Non-immune hydrops fetalis

A 34-year-old Caucasian, para 7 + 0 woman attended the antenatal booking clinic at 12 weeks' gestation. She had conceived whilst awaiting a laparoscopic sterilization and had decided to continue with the pregnancy. Her seven previous pregnancies had been uncomplicated, and each had ended with the vaginal delivery of an appropriately grown baby. Her blood group was A rhesus positive, and no antibodies had been detected in previous pregnancies. She was a smoker, and was advised to discontinue; her past medical history was otherwise unremarkable. An ultrasound scan indicated that the fetal size was consistent with her last menstrual period. In view of her grand multiparity, the management plan was for intravenous access in labour with her serum to be grouped and saved for cross matching.

A routine 20-week fetal anomaly scan noted a large pleural effusion and gross abdominal ascites – the fetal stomach could not be visualized. She was referred to a fetal medicine specialist who repeated the ultrasound scan; the previous findings of gross fetal hydrops were confirmed, a large left-sided hydrothorax was seen, with consequent displacement and rotation of a normal-sized heart, which had a normal internal structure. The fetal heart rate was normal and regular.

QI: **What are the ultrasonographic criteria for a diagnosis of fetal hydrops?**

Q2: **Which of the following are causes of non-immune fetal hydrops?**
A: Parvovirus BI9 infection.
B: Turner's syndrome.
C: Antibodies to K in the Kell system.
D: Fallot's tetralogy.
E: Osteogenesis imperfecta.
F: Congenital nephrosis.

Q3: **What are the other major causes of non-immune fetal hydrops?**

A maternal blood sample was taken.

Q4: **What investigations would you perform on the maternal blood sample?**

Q5: **When counselling the patient, which of the following statements regarding non-immune fetal hydrops are true?**
A: Reported fetal mortality rates are approximately 30%.
B: The prognosis deteriorates with increasing gestational age at diagnosis.

C: Treatment can be offered in the majority of cases.

D: Maternal risks include an increased incidence of pre-eclampsia.

All investigations of the maternal blood sample were negative. After counselling, it was suggested that fetal blood sampling should be performed and that the hydrothorax should be drained. However, the patient was adamant that she did not wish any invasive procedures to be performed. She was not prepared to contemplate a termination of pregnancy under any circumstances.

Q6: What would have been the advantage of fetal blood sampling?

Q7: What would have been the advantage of draining the hydrothorax?

The patient reattended the antenatal clinic at 27 weeks' gestation and remained asymptomatic. On examination, the symphysis fundal height was 41 cm and the lie was thought to be longitudinal, although it was difficult to palpate fetal parts due to clinical polyhydramnios. An ultrasound scan revealed gross fetal hydrops, with bilateral pleural effusions, skin oedema and abdominal ascites. The biparietal diameter was 75 mm (equivalent to 29 weeks' gestation) and the abdominal circumference was 394 mm (equivalent to term+). Polyhydramnios was confirmed; the maximum pool of liquor was 13 cm. The placenta was noted to be covering the os. The grave prognosis was reiterated and the patient was advised to attend the labour ward if she noted any contractions or vaginal bleeding.

At 28+ weeks' gestation, she was admitted to the labour ward following a small antepartum haemorrhage (less than a teaspoonful of blood). The findings on examination were unchanged. Four units of blood were cross-matched and she was admitted to the antenatal ward. An ultrasound scan the following day indicated a grade IV placenta praevia, and a breech presentation was noted. The abdominal circumference was above the median for a term fetus. The patient then reported irregular uterine activity, and it was decided to perform a Caesarean section.

At lower segment Caesarean section, marked polyhydramnios was noted. A female infant, weighing 1.98 kg, with a grossly distended abdomen, was delivered to the awaiting paediatricians. A hydropic placenta weighing 1.3 kg was delivered. There was minimal bleeding from the placental bed, and the operation was uncomplicated. Despite drainage of bilateral hydrothoraces and of ascites (a total of 500 ml was removed), resuscitation was difficult. Apgar scores of 2 at 1 minute, 2 at 5 minutes, 2 at 10 minutes and 5 at 15 minutes were recorded. The infant was transferred to the special care baby unit, ventilated, at 25 minutes of age. Ventilation was continued using high pressures in 95% oxygen. Despite this, the infant's oxygen ~ation remained below 50%. The right chest was reaspirated but fluid was obtained. A chest radiograph showed severe pulmonary and subcutaneous oedema with probable hyaline membrane ial blood gases showed a severe respiratory and metabolic acidosis with a pH of 6.77 and a base excess of -19.1 mEq l^{-1}. At 5 hours of age, the infant was obviously making poor progress and, after discussion with her parents, the decision to withdraw intensive care was taken.

A subsequent post-mortem examination revealed a large right-sided congenital diaphragmatic hernia, with liver within the fetal chest. The liver was rotated, with occlusion of the ductus venosus. This was presumably the cause of the fetal hydrops, via occlusion of venous return to the heart. The fetal lung volumes were greatly diminished: 10 and 14 ml in the left and right lungs respectively.

> **Q8: Which of the following statements concerning congenital diaphragmatic hernia are correct?**
> A: The diaphragm normally forms between 4 and 8 weeks' gestation.
> B: The incidence is approximately 1:3000 live births.
> C: The defect is usually unilateral and on the right side.
> D: Mortality rate is between 50 and 80%
>
> **Q9: Why do you think that the diagnosis was missed on ultrasound scan?**

The maternal postoperative recovery was unremarkable, and the patient subsequently underwent a laparoscopic clip sterilization.

COMMENTARY

Fetal hydrops is diagnosed when ultrasonography shows generalized skin oedema (greater than 5 mm) and collections of fluid in visceral cavities (pleural effusion, pericardial effusion or ascites). If only one serous cavity is involved, the presence of an abnormally thick placenta is also required for the diagnosis. The ratio of non-immune to immune hydrops is about 9:1, and the incidence of non-immune hydrops is approximately 1:1000 births (**Q1**).

Over 70 causes of non-immune fetal hydrops have been reported, the majority of which are rare. One or more of the following mechanisms is involved in all of these causes:

- Inadequate cardiac output: due to obstructed or diverted outflow, deficient cardiac return or insufficient ionotropic force.
- Decreased plasma oncotic pressure.
- Increased capillary permeability.
- Obstruction of lymphatic flow.

Parvovirus infection classically presents as fetal hydrops, due to either anaemia, myocarditis or hepatitis. Chromosomal anomalies account for a significant number of cases of non-immune hydrops; the most common anomalies are trisomies, Turner's syndrome (45XO), and triploidy. vere congenital heart disease (such as Fallot's tetralogy) is a recognize e of hydrops, as are renal malformations including congenital nephrosis. Anti-Kell antibodies could result in immune hydrops fetalis. Osteogenesis imperfecta is not a cause of fetal hydrops (**Q2: true = A, B, D, F; false = C, E**).

Most cases of non-immune fetal hydrops fall into one of nine major categories (Table 1). In all series, there are cases in which no cause is found. The proportion of 'idiopathic' hydrops depends on the vigour with which a diagnosis is pursued (**Q3**).

Whenever fetal hydrops is diagnosed, a maternal red cell antibody screen should be performed to exclude isoimmune disease. A large number of other tests have been suggested to diagnose other causes. Most of these

TABLE I MAJOR CATEGORIES OF NON-IMMUNE HYDROPS FETALIS	
Cause	**Approximate percentage of cases**
Chromosomal abnormality Trisomies, Turner's syndrome, triploidy	20
Cardiovascular malformations Severe congenital heart disease, premature closure of foramen ovale/ductus, large arteriovenous malformations	20
Cardiac arrhythmias Tachycardias, bradycardias, Wolff–Parkinson–White syndrome	15
Anaemia α-Thalassaemia, fetomaternal transfusion, twin–twin transfusion	15
Malformation syndromes Pulmonary (cystic adenomatous malformation, diaphragmatic hernia) Renal (congenital nephrosis, renal vein thrombosis) Cystic hygroma	15
Infections Parvovirus, cytomegalovirus, toxoplasmosis, herpes simplex, syphilis, leptospirosis	10
Liver disease Calcification, fibrosis, congenital hepatitis, cholestasis, metabolic storage diseases	5
Miscellaneous Achondroplasia, tuberous sclerosis, sacrococcygeal teratoma	5
Idiopathic	10

have a very low yield, as the diseases they screen for are most uncommon. For example, most authors recommend a Kleihauer test, even though a fetomaternal haemorrhage is a rare cause of non-immune hydrops. Tests may include a full blood count, serology for syphilis, parvovirus, cytomegalovirus, coxsackie, herpes simplex and toxoplasmosis, and tests of glucose tolerance. Depending on the ethnic and genetic background of the patient, haemoglobin electrophoresis to detect α-thalassaemia carrier status or tests for glucose-6-phosphate dehydrogenase or pyruvate kinase levels in maternal red blood cells may be done (**Q4**).

The overall mortality rate is about 80% in most series. Features associated with a poor prognosis include the coexistence of malformations, large pleural effusions (which result in pulmonary hypoplasia), progressive ascites and oedema, and an early gestational age at diagnosis. α-Thalassaemias and some cardiac malformations are invariably fatal. The best prognosis is associated with fetal arrhythmias, which may respond to pharmacological intervention. Other cases are potentially treatable; hydrops associated with other causes of inadequate cardiac output (anaemia, hydrothoraces, recipient in twin–twin transfusions) have been treated by *in utero* transfusion and chronic shunt placement. Pre-eclampsia has been reported to occur in up to 40% of cases and may necessitate premature delivery (**Q5: true = D; false = A, B, C**).

Fetal blood sampling would have enabled determination of the fetal karyotype, a full blood count (including haemoglobin concentration), serological tests for IgM antibodies for infection, liver enzymes and blood gas determination. In addition, measurement of the intravascular pressure allows rapid separation of cardiac and non-cardiac causes of fetal hydrops. Abnormal pressure almost excludes a cardiac cause, whereas a raised pressure is strongly suggestive of cardiac disease (**Q6**). If the fetal heart is displaced from the normal midline position by a pleural effusion, most authors recommend that the fetal chest should be punctured, the intrathoracic pressure measured, and the effusion drained (Weiner, 1993). The benefits of this therapy are unproven; it is well recognized that the fluid rapidly reaccumulates (**Q7**).

During embryonic development, the muscular diaphragm forms between 6 and 14 weeks' gestation as a result of a complicated chain of events involving the fusion of four structures: the septum transversum, the pleuroperitoneal membranes, the dorsal mesentery of the oesophagus, and the body wall. The incidence of failure of this fusion, and thus development of a diaphragmatic hernia, is between 1:2000 and 1:5000 live births. The defect is usually unilateral (97%) and on the left (75–90%). The mortality rate associated with diaphragmatic hernia is high (50–80%), and polyhydramnios is an especially poor prognostic indicator (**Q8: true = B, D; false = A, C**).

Right-sided hernias are less common. Although there may be associated suggestive findings, such as hydrothorax and ascites, right-sided lesions are more difficult to identify owing to the similar echogenicity of the liver and lungs. Identification of the gallbladder in the chest may be a useful ancillary finding in confirming the diagnosis in these cases (**Q9**).

REFERENCE

Weiner CP. Umbilical pressure measurement in the evaluation of nonimmune hydrops fetalis. *Am J Obstet Gynecol* 1993; **168**: 817–823.

FACTS YOU SHOULD HAVE LEARNT . . .

▶ The incidence, definition and diagnosis of hydrops fetalis
▶ The differential diagnosis and pathogenesis of hydrops fetalis
▶ The appropriate investigations in hydrops fetalis

CASE 3

Recurrent pregnancy loss

A 26-year-old para 1 + 2 Caucasian woman attended the antenatal booking clinic at 8 weeks' gestation. She had a complex past medical history. She had suffered two first trimester miscarriages 5 and 3 years previously. In both cases there had been no evidence of an embryo. Her third pregnancy had been uneventful until she presented at 28 weeks' gestation with an intrauterine fetal death. A 723 g stillborn, growth-restricted, male infant was delivered after an induced labour. The placenta had contained focal infarctions. Following her third pregnancy, lupus anticoagulant was identified, and a diagnosis of antiphospholipid syndrome was made.

Q1: **Which other thrombotic coagulopathies could result in the above history of recurrent fetal loss?**
A: Klippel–Trenaunay–Weber syndrome.
B: Protein C deficiency.
C: Deficiency of plasminogen activator inhibitor.
D: Paroxysmal nocturnal haemoglobinuria.
E: Antithrombin III deficiency.

Q2: **What is antiphospholipid syndrome?**

Q3: **How is lupus anticoagulant identified?**

Q4: **Which of the following are indications for investigation of antiphospholipid syndrome?**
A: Autoimmune disorders, such as systemic lupus erythematosus.
B: A false-positive VDRL (Venereal Disease Reference Laboratory) test.
C: Severe, early onset or recurrent pre-eclampsia.
D: Recurrent first- or second-trimester miscarriages.
E: Molar pregnancies.
F: Raised maternal serum α-fetoprotein.

Q5: **What investigations should be performed in patients found to have antiphospholipid syndrome?**

Findings on examination were unremarkable. An ultrasound scan confirmed the presence of a viable fetus.

Q6: **When considering management during pregnancy, which of the following statements are correct?**
A: Maximal benefits are achieved if therapy is started before conception.
B: A combination of prednisolone and low-dose aspirin has been shown to improve outcome.

C: Subcutaneous heparin therapy has been shown to improve outcome.
D: The majority of patients with antiphospholipid syndrome deliver before
32 weeks' gestation.

The patient was commenced on low molecular weight heparin
10 000 IU daily, and at 13 weeks' gestation low-dose aspirin was prescribed.

Q7: **Which of the following are complications of low molecular weight
heparin therapy for several months during pregnancy?**
A: Clinically overt osteoporosis in less than 5% of patients.
B: Thrombocytopenia in approximately 20% of patients.
C: Fetal central nervous system abnormalities in 2–3% of cases.
D: Fetal intracranial haemorrhage at the time of delivery.

Q8: **How would you monitor low molecular weight heparin therapy?**

At 20 weeks' gestation, the dose of low molecular weight heparin was
increased to 15 000 IU daily. An ultrasound scan at 24 weeks' gestation
demonstrated a normal liquor volume, but fetal measurements that were
compatible with only 22 weeks' gestation. Serial ultrasound scans at 27
and 30 weeks' gestation indicated that both head circumference and
abdominal circumference measurements were below the 5th centile (the
estimated fetal weight at 30 weeks' gestation was 900 g). Biophysical profile
scores at 28 and 29 weeks' gestation were 8 and 10 respectively. However,
at 30 weeks' gestation, the biophysical profile score was 4, with no fetal
breathing, diminished liquor volume and no fetal movements. The
biophysical profile is discussed further in case 16.

On vaginal examination the cervix was closed and it was decided to
perform a Caesarean section. Heparin therapy was discontinued and
dexamethasone was administered intramuscularly. At lower segment
Caesarean section the following day, a male infant weighing 935 g was
born with an Apgar score of 8 at 1 minute and of 9 at 5 minutes.
Umbilical artery blood gas analysis included a pH of 7.31 and a base excess
of -2.3 mEq l^{-1}. The infant had mild respiratory distress but no other
significant neonatal complications. The 180 g placenta was histologically
normal apart from a peripheral infarct 2 cm in diameter.

The patient's postoperative course was uncomplicated. Warfarin was
commenced immediately after delivery, although heparin prophylaxis was
continued for 4 days until the INR (international normalized ratio) was
2.0.

COMMENTARY

Klippel–Trenaunay–Weber syndrome is not a thrombotic coagulopathy; it
involves bony and soft tissue hypertrophy in combination with venous
varicosity, and is often confined to a single limb. Protein C is a vitamin K-
dependent plasma protein, which, when activated, inhibits the ability of

activated factors V and VIII to facilitate clot formation. Deficiencies in protein C (and protein S, which is a co-factor for activated protein C) have been reported in early-onset growth restriction and pre-eclampsia, and in third-trimester stillbirths. Fibrinolytic activity is reduced in normal pregnancy due to placentally derived plasminogen activator inhibitors. A deficiency of plasminogen activator inhibitors would increase fibrinolytic activity. Paroxysmal nocturnal haemoglobinuria is a manifestation of an unusual susceptibility to lysis by complement. Often cases are discovered in the course of investigating chronic iron deficiency anaemia. Women with paroxysmal nocturnal haemoglobinuria are often infertile; if they conceive, spontaneous abortion and intrauterine death are commonplace. Antithrombin III is an α_2-globulin which regulates coagulation by inhibiting active forms of vitamin K-dependent clotting factors, and antithrombin II deficiency has also been implicated in recurrent fetal loss (**Q1: true = B, D, E; false = A, C**).

Antiphospholipid syndrome is an autoimmune condition characterized by antiphospholipid antibodies (lupus anticoagulant and anticardiolipin antibodies) and certain clinical features including thrombotic disease (arterial or venous), autoimmune thrombocytopenia and pregnancy loss. The antibodies react with phospholipids on platelets or endothelial cell membranes, causing platelet and vascular damage, which in turn results in thromboembolic disorders and placental malfunction, the common clinical manifestations of the syndrome. Lupus anticoagulant also interferes with prostacyclin production, which may account for the high incidence of pre-eclampsia noted in these women (**Q2**).

The term 'lupus anticoagulant' is a double misnomer because it is neither an anticoagulant *in vivo* nor exclusively associated with lupus erythematosus. There is considerable debate as to the most reliable method of screening for, and confirming the presence of, lupus anticoagulant. The most common screening test is the activated partial thromboplastin time (APTT). If the APTT is prolonged and cannot be corrected to a normal mixture with an admixture of normal plasma 1:1, a circulating anticoagulant must be suspected. The kaolin clotting time (KCT) is one of the more sensitive methods of confirming the presence of lupus anticoagulant. In contrast, anticardiolipin antibody can be directly demonstrated by reaction with its specific antigen. The simplest test for the presence of anticardiolipin antibody is the VDRL test which uses cardiolipin as antigen. More recently described radioimmunoassays and enzyme immunoassays offer greater sensitivity (**Q3**).

Indications for the investigation of women in obstetric populations for the antiphospholipid syndrome include recurrent fetal loss (in any trimester), severe intrauterine growth restriction, autoimmune disorders (such as systemic lupus erythematosus), arterial or venous thromboembolic events, severe, early-onset or recurrent pre-eclampsia, thrombocytopenia, pulmonary hypertension, chorea gravidarum, a false-positive VDRL test, or a first-degree relative with antiphospholipid syndrome (**Q4: true = A, B, C, D; false = E, F**).

It is important that all patients found to have antiphospholipid syndrome should also be investigated for associated autoimmune disorders; there is a particularly strong association with systemic lupus erythematosus. The requisite tests: antinuclear antibody (ANA), anti-DNA antibody, complement levels, a test for circulating immune complexes and organ-specific autoantibodies, should all be performed. Patients should be tested for anti-Ro antibodies as congenital heart block may develop in fetuses whose mothers are anti-Ro positive. Patients with antiphospholipid syndrome, like those with systemic lupus erythematosus, should be assessed for underlying evidence of anaemia, thrombocytopenia and renal disease (urinalysis, serum creatinine, 24-hour urine collection for protein estimation and creatinine clearance) (**Q5**).

There is evidence that treatment in early pregnancy is beneficial, but there is no such evidence to suggest that starting this therapy before conception improves outcome. The majority of studies on the effect of prednisolone and low-dose aspirin have been uncontrolled. Nevertheless, almost all authors have concluded that this combination is beneficial. There have been fewer studies of the effect of heparin therapy for patients with antiphospholipid syndrome. These studies suggest that subcutaneous heparin, with or without low-dose aspirin, has a similar beneficial effect. Treatment with either glucocorticoids and low-dose aspirin, or heparin and low-dose aspirin, does not seem to reduce the incidence of preterm delivery, which approximates to 30% of women with antiphospholipid syndrome delivering before 32 weeks' gestation (**Q6: true = B, C; false = A, D**).

None of the low molecular weight heparins is licensed for use in pregnancy; however, following publication of Royal College of Obstetricians and Gynaecologists' guidelines (RCOG Working Party, 1995), use of this therapy has become common practice in the UK. Advantages of low molecular weight heparin include a lower incidence of osteoporosis and thrombocytopenia when compared with the use of unfractionated heparin therapy (complication rates of less than 5% and 2–3% respectively). As heparin does not cross the placenta, teratogenic effects (typical of warfarin therapy) are not seen (**Q7: False=A, B, C, D**). Anti-X_a should be measured monthly, aiming to achieve levels of 0.2–0.4 IU ml^{-1} 4–6 hours after injection (**Q8**).

REFERENCE

RCOG Working Party. *Report of the RCOG Working Party on Prophylaxis against Thromboembolism in Gynaecology and Obstetrics.* London: RCOG Press, 1995.

FACTS YOU SHOULD HAVE LEARNT . . .

▶ Thrombotic coagulopathies that can result in recurrent fetal loss
▶ The diagnosis, pathogenesis and complications of antiphospholipid syndrome
▶ The management of antiphospholipid syndrome
▶ The use of low molecular weight heparin in pregnancy
▶ The characteristics and implications of the biophysical profile

CASE 4

Excessive nausea and vomiting

A 29-year-old married Pakistani P0 + 0 woman was admitted to hospital with a 10-day history of nausea and vomiting. She had no significant past medical history and was approximately 9 weeks' pregnant. She did not drink alcohol and was not a vegetarian. On examination she looked unwell and appeared clinically dehydrated and her breath smelt ketotic. Her temperature was 37°C, her pulse was 88 beats per minute (bpm) and her blood pressure was 90/55 mmHg. Her abdomen was soft and non-tender.

> **Q1: What investigations would you perform to establish the diagnosis and why would you perform them?**

Urinalysis revealed 3+ ketones and no protein, sugar, blood or urobilinogen.

> **Q2: Which of the following treatment/s should be instituted whilst awaiting the results of your investigations?**
> A: Metoclopramide 10 mg intramuscularly every 4 hours as required.
> B: Rehydration with 10% dextrose and commence an insulin infusion.
> C: Rehydration with 5% dextrose and/or 0.9% saline solution.
> D: Amoxycillin 500 mg intravenously every 8 hours.
> E: Rehydration with 0.9% saline solution with potassium chloride additive.
> F: Oral carbimazole 5 mg once daily.

> **Q3: Which of the following statements are correct?**
> A: At 9 weeks' gestation organogenesis is complete, therefore antiemetics are safe to use.
> B: Gastro-oesopheal reflux is a common and potent cause of nausea and vomiting in the first trimester of pregnancy.
> C: The patient may have hypokalaemic alkalosis.
> D: The patient should be catheterized to monitor urine output as she is at risk of developing acute tubular necrosis.
> E: A gastroscopy should be arranged to exclude gastric ulceration and *Helicobacter pylori* infection.

The early results of your investigations showed the following: Na 145 mmol l^{-1}, K 3.0 mmol l^{-1}, urea 1.0 µmol l^{-1}, creatinine 50 µmol l^{-1}, haemoglobin 13.2 g dl^{-1}, platelets 200 × 10^9 l^{-1}, white cell count 10 × 10^9 l^{-1} with a normal distribution, red cell indices normal apart from a mean corpuscular volume of 110 fl.

Q4: Which of the following statements about red cell macrocytosis are correct?
A: It can be either megaloblastic or normoblastic on bone marrow biopsy.
B: It can be caused by both vitamin B_{12} and folate deficiency.
C: It may be caused by pregnancy.
D: Causes include thyrotoxicosis, liver disease and alcohol consumption.
E: All cases associated with anaemia should be investigated.

After rehydration, the patient's condition improved and her urine output was satisfactory with no evidence of ketosis. She continued to feel nauseated and to vomit, and requested something to make her feel better.

Q5: Which, if any, antiemetic drug would you prescribe?

Three hours after the administration of 12.5 mg prochlorperazine, the patient had 'a funny turn' or fit. She was conscious and responded to commands but was rigid, her teeth were clenched and she had a fixed upward gaze.

Q6: Which of the following are possible diagnoses?
A: Hypokalaemic paralysis.
B: Hypoglycaemia.
C: Sagittal sinus thrombosis.
D: Occulogyric crisis.
E: Wernicke's encephalopathy.
F: Subacute combined degeneration.

Q7: What treatment should you offer immediately?

The next day she had recovered but the nausea and vomiting continued and the serum levels of electrolytes are normal. Thyroid function test results were as follows: free thyroxine 28 pmol l^{-1} (normal 10–20 pmol l^{-1}), thyroid stimulating hormone (TSH) < 0.1 mIU l^{-1} (normal 0.1–5.5 mIU l^{-1}), T3 3.6 pmol l^{-1} (normal 3.5–6.5 pmol l^{-1}).

Q8: What other tests would you order to investigate the possible thyroid dysfunction?

The patient was commenced on carbimazole 20 mg at night. The thyroid microsomal antibodies were negative indicating no evidence of thyroid cell breakdown. In addition, no auto-immune antibodies to intrinsic factor and parietal cells were detected.

Q9: Which of the following statements about carbimazole in pregnancy are correct?
A: Its use is contraindicated.
B: It can cause aplasia cutis in the fetus.
C: It can cause skin rashes in the woman.

D: It can cause neutropenia.

E: At this gestation, it crosses the placenta, enters the fetal circulation and suppresses fetal thyroid function.

The patient's symptoms improved and she was discharged.

Q10: What follow-up would you arrange and what advice would you give to her?

Q11: What other treatments have been used successfully in cases of intractable hyperemesis gravidarum?

The patient's symptoms settled and she was discharged home. She was followed up in the antenatal clinic with monthly thyroid function tests. The antithyroid medications were stopped at 24 weeks' gestation and thyroid function test results remained normal. All investigations related to the red cell macrocytosis were negative.

COMMENTARY

This patient's 10-day history of nausea and vomiting necessitated that her urine should be analysed for ketones, protein, blood and a sample sent for culture to exclude urinary tract infection. You should have arranged for serum electrolytes, renal function and liver function tests to be performed as these may all be abnormal as a result of the vomiting and dehydration. A full blood count would help determine any possible vitamin deficiency and give an assessment of the degree of dehydration (this would result in a raised haemoglobin concentration and packed cell volume). Thyroid function tests should be performed to exclude Graves' disease. Human chorionic gonadotrophin (hCG) can bind to the TSH receptor on the thyroid gland and stimulate endogenous thyroxine synthesis and secretion (Vanderpump *et al*, 1996). An ultrasound scan will confirm an intrauterine pregnancy and diagnose pregnancies with hyperplacentosis (e.g. multiple pregnancy and hydatidiform moles) (**Q1**).

Treatment should commence to correct dehydration, electrolyte disturbances and ketosis. Generally 0.9% saline is the fluid of choice with 5% dextrose to reverse the ketosis to prevent oliguria. Too much dextrose will produce hyponatraemia, which is dangerous, especially in the presence of water-soluble vitamin deficiency (Bergin and Harvey, 1992). Other treatments should be commenced only with specific proof of abnormality. Anti-emetic therapy should be withheld until dehydration and ketosis have been corrected (**Q2: true = C; false = A, B, D, E, F**).

At 9 weeks' gestation organogenesis is not complete (brain, eyes, ears, teeth, external genitalia). Antiemetics are contraindicated in pregnancy according to the drug safety literature, although the evidence that they increase the risk of structural congenital abnormalities above and beyond that seen in the human species (3%) is weak. Gastro-oesophageal reflux is a common and potent cause of nausea and vomiting in pregnancy, but usually in the second and third trimesters. A history of dyspepsia in the pre-pregnant state should alert the gynaecologist to the possibility of gastric ulceration and in such cases a gastroscopy should be arranged to exclude peptic ulceration and *H. pylori* infection. At this stage there is no need to catheterize the patient to monitor urine output. However, if oliguria is present then the patient is at risk of developing acute tubular necrosis and renal failure; this was the main cause of death in past times. Hypokalaemic alkalosis may develop with vomiting and thus you should not administer Hartmann's solution which contains lactate and bicarbonate, and may exacerbate any pH disturbance (**Q3: true = C; false = A, B, D, E**).

Patients with red cell macrocytosis can be found to have megaloblastic bone marrow as a consequence of vitamin B_{12} and folate deficiency, from malabsorption syndromes, dietary deficiencies and pregnancy. However, the bone marrow may be normoblastic as a consequence of myxoedema, liver disease, alcohol consumption and myeloproliferative disorders. Red cell macrocytosis should thus be investigated in all cases (Bergin and Harvey, 1992). In this case the red cell macrocytosis should alert you to the distinct possibility of vitamin deficiencies; folate, vitamin B_{12} and thiamine deficiency should be considered (**Q4: true = A, B, C, E; false = D**).

A dopamine antagonist may be prescribed to help relieve the symptoms of nausea and vomiting. They suppress pro-emetic stimuli by blocking the D_2 receptors in the chemoreceptor trigger zone. The common drugs used are metoclopramide 10 mg and prochlorperazine 12.5 mg intramuscularly, 6 hourly as required. The disadvantages are that they also block dopamine receptors elsewhere in the brain, particularly the nigrostriatal pathway which may produce extrapyramidal reactions. Domperidone (5 mg intramuscularly 6 hourly) does not readily cross the blood–brain barrier and is theoretically less likely to cause extrapyramidal problems. 5-hydroxytryptamine antagonists (granisetron, ondansetron, tropisetron) do not cause extrapyramidal side-effects and have potent actions; however, they are not commonly used in pregnancy and are contraindicated in the drug safety literature (**Q5**).

In this case the most likely diagnosis is an occulogyric crisis. Sagittal sinus thrombosis is a possibility in view of the vomiting, which is a common symptom, but the condition is often associated with loss of consciousness. Wernicke's encepholopathy is a distinct possibility; generally it is associated with bilateral VI cranial nerve palsy, confusion and loss of consciousness. Thiamine (20 mg at night) should be administered to woman with severe prolonged hyperemesis (Bergin and Harvey, 1992). Subacute combined degeneration of the spinal columns and peripheral neuropathy are associated with vitamin B_{12} deficiency and the signs are demonstrated mainly in the lower limbs. Hypokalaemic paralysis and hypoglycaemia are not likely (**Q6: true = D, perhaps C, E; false = A, B, F**).

The patient needed an anticholinergic drug to treat this acute dystonia. The drug of choice is benztropine mesylate 1–2 mg intravenously. The cure is instantaneous (**Q7**).

The other test required to investigate the possibility of Graves' disease was quantification of thyroid microsomal antibodies (otherwise known as thyroid peroxidase antibodies) in the serum. This will establish the cause for the thyroid dysfunction (usually a titre greater than 1/1600 is significant). In view of the possible autoimmune cause of the red cell macrocytosis, determination of autoantibodies to intrinsic factor and parietal cells should be considered. The assumption that this is a pregnancy-related thyrotoxicosis episode means that treatment should cure the patient's symptoms. There are two options: propylthiouracil 100 mg (given at night to maximize chances of absorption) or carbimazole 5–20 mg at night (**Q8**).

Carbimazole is not contraindicated in pregnancy but should be used with caution. It can cause aplasia cutis in the fetus but this is a rare side-effect. Carbimazole can cause skin rashes and neutropenia. It does cross the placenta, enters the fetal circulation and suppresses fetal thyroid function later in pregnancy but not at this gestation (**Q9: true = B, C, D; false = A, E**).

Following any such episode, patients should be followed up in the antenatal clinic with monthly thyroid function tests. Antithyroid medication can be stopped in the second trimester in cases not thought to be due to autoimmune-related thyrotoxicosis. Thyroid function tests should be repeated at the postnatal visit to confirm the pregnancy-related nature of the thyrotoxicosis. Patients started on carbimazole should be warned to consult their doctor if a rash develops or they develop a sore throat. The drug should be suspended and a full blood count performed. With this patient's propensity to extrapyramidal side-effects from antiemetics at relatively low doses, caution should be exhibited in labour if opiates and antiemetics are contemplated (**Q10**).

In cases of intractable hyperemesis gravidarum, case reports support the use of high-dose prednisolone (40 mg per day) (Nelson-Piercy and de Swiet, 1994). It is important to exclude peptic ulceration of the upper gastrointestinal tract before commencement. Other therapeutic options include total parenteral nutrition and occasionally even termination of pregnancy (**Q11**).

REFERENCES

Bergin PS, Harvey P. Wernicke's encephalopathy and central pontine myelinolysis associated with hyperemesis gravidarum. *BMJ* 1992; **305**: 517–518.

Nelson-Piercy C, de Swiet M. Corticosteroids for the treatment of hyperemesis gravidarum. *Br J Obstet Gynaecol* 1994; **101**: 1013–1015.

Vanderpump MPJ, Ahlquist JAO, Franklyn JA, Clayton RN. Consensus statement for good practice and audit measures in the management of hypothyroidism and hyperthyroidism. *BMJ* 1996; **313**: 539–544.

FACTS YOU SHOULD HAVE LEANRT . . .

▶ The differential diagnosis and management of hyperemesis gravidarum
▶ The management of an oculogyric crisis
▶ The management of thyroid dysfunction in pregnancy

CASE 5

Ectopic pregnancy

A 25-year-old woman presented to her general practitioner with a 2-day history of lower abdominal pain. The pain was more marked on the right side and went into her back. She had vomited on several occasions. Paracetamol had had little effect. She had used the progestogen-only pill for contraception and had irregular periods with a light bleed only. Her last bleed had occurred 1 week earlier.

On examination she had a temperature of 37.3°C, her pulse was 90 bpm with a blood pressure of 110/70 mmHg. On palpation, she was tender in the right iliac fossa with no guarding. On vaginal assessment there was no significant discharge. The cervix looked healthy. The uterus was anteverted, mobile and not tender. There was some discomfort in both fornices, more marked on the right side.

Q1: Which of the following should be included in your differential diagnosis?
A: Appendicitis.
B: Pelvic inflammatory disease.
C: Cholecystitis.
D: Urinary tract infection.
E: Ectopic pregnancy.

Q2: Which of the following investigations would you instigate?
A: Abdominal radiography.
B: Human chorionic gonadotrophin (hCG) assay.
C: Serum amylase.
D: Pelvic ultrasonography.
E: Urine culture.

The patient was given co-proxamol (dextropropoxyphene hydrochoride and paracetamol) for pain, which was effective. Her haemoglobin level was 11.7 gm dl^{-1}. The pregnancy test was weakly positive. An ultrasound scan of the pelvis showed a uterus containing a small sac without any evidence of a fetus. There was some free fluid in the pouch of Douglas and the ovaries were normal.

She remained in hospital for 24 hours during which time the pain settled. She was sent home with an appointment to return for an ultrasound scan in 2 weeks' time.

Q3: Do you consider that this management was appropriate?

The urine culture and triple swabs were negative. Six days later, the patient was readmitted with increasing pain and more vaginal bleeding.

The latter was not heavy, but the pain was more intense than before with the same location. On examination, she had a temperature of 37.4°C, a pulse of 96 bpm and a blood pressure of 110/60 mmHg. She was very tender in the right iliac fossa with localized guarding. A pregnancy test remained positive and an ultrasound scan was similar to the previous one, although the intrauterine sac was a little larger than before but no fetal pole was identified.

Co-proxamol was not fully effective for control of the pain, but one dose of pethidine settled the symptoms.

Q4: What are the management options?

Assays for hCG from the two pregnancy tests revealed the following levels:

First admission 50 IU ml^{-1}
Second admission 180 IU ml^{-1}

It was thought that the patient might have an early intrauterine pregnancy. The decision was made to manage her conservatively and check the hCG assay again in 48 hours. The pain became worse during the 24 hours after admission and she required regular injections of pethidine to control it. The observations remained stable.

In view of the worsening symptoms, a decision was made to perform a laparoscopy with consent to proceed if an ectopic pregnancy was diagnosed.

At operation, she was found to have a small volume of blood in the pouch of Douglas with a 3-cm right-sided ampullary ectopic pregnancy. The left tube and both ovaries appeared normal.

A laparoscopic salpingotomy was performed by operating on the tube with diathermy and sucking out the contents of the sac.

Q5: Would you have performed a salpingectomy or salpingotomy?

Q6: How would you follow up the patient?

The woman made a good recovery. She attended the outpatient clinic 6 weeks later. She had had a normal period the week before and had just started taking the combined oral contraceptive pill.

Q7: How would you counsel her regarding further pregnancies?

COMMENTARY

The location of the pain at presentation made the diagnosis of cholecystitis unlikely. The other possible problems should all have been considered. Whilst she had had a bleed 1 week earlier, this does not exclude an ectopic pregnancy as such bleeding may mimic a normal period. It is also not unusual to have mild pyrexia associated with tubal pregnancy, particularly if there has been some intraperitoneal bleeding (**Q1: true = A, B, D, E; false = C**).

The investigations of choice would be a full blood count, a hCG assay, urine culture, vaginal and cervical swabs, and pelvic ultrasonography. A vaginal ultrasound probe gives better details of the pelvis although failure to observe an adnexal mass does not exclude tubal pregnancy. The uterus enlarges in response to any pregnancy and the observation of a possible gestation sac on ultrasonography may be confused with a pseudogestational sac within the uterine cavity (**Q2: true = B, D, E; false = A, C**).

Although the woman's pain settled over the 24 hours after admission, there were risks in sending her home as tubal pregnancy had not been categorically excluded. It was particularly dangerous not to review her for 2 weeks. Ideally, the hCG assay should have been quantified and a repeat level measured 48 hours later. In the presence of a continuing intrauterine pregnancy, the second assay should have increased by at least 66% (Kadar *et al*, 1981). Failure of such an increase should have prompted readmission and probable laparoscopy (**Q3**).

When the patient was readmitted 6 days later the situation was very suspicious of an ectopic pregnancy, particularly as there was little change in the ultrasonographic appearance of the uterus. The management options at this stage were either laparoscopy to confirm or exclude an ectopic pregnancy, or inpatient monitoring of hCG levels. In view of the fact that she required pethidine to control the pain, the authors would have advised immediate diagnostic laparoscopy – the risk of an ectopic pregnancy was great and the risk of waiting was rupture with serious intraperitoneal bleeding. The increase in the hCG level between admissions was at the very lower end of what might have been expected with an intrauterine pregnancy (**Q4**).

When the patient was finally taken to theatre, the diagnosis of a right-sided tubal pregnancy was made and a decision was taken to perform salpingotomy rather than salpingectomy. There has been a considerable amount of literature relating to both the subsequent risk of ectopic pregnancy as well as the likelihood of a successful intrauterine pregnancy occurring. It would appear that the state of the contralateral tube is the most important factor relating to the risk of a future ectopic pregnancy (Ory *et al*, 1993). There is a slightly increased risk of further ectopic pregnancy following salpingotomy rather than salpingectomy, and salpingotomy should probably be reserved for cases where the other tube is obviously damaged or absent (**Q5**).

Following salpingotomy, there is a risk of trophoblastic tissue persisting and proliferating. It is therefore important after such a procedure to monitor the hCG level over a few days to make sure that it is falling. This can be done as an outpatient investigation so long as the woman is symptom free (**Q6**).

Having had an ectopic pregnancy, this woman would be at increased risk of a further one. This relates not only to the fact that the commonest aetiological factor is intrinsic tubal damage, which is usually bilateral, but also to the fact that conservative surgery with tubal preservation was undertaken for this pregnancy. You should warn her of the increased risk of repeat tubal pregnancy and advise her to present early in any subsequent pregnancy for confirmation of an intrauterine location. She should probably be advised against the risk of an intrauterine contraceptive device. She should also be reassured that the chance of a subsequent intrauterine pregnancy occurring is good, particularly as the contralateral tube looked normal at the time of laparoscopy (**Q7**).

REFERENCES

Kadar N, De Vore G, Romero R. Discriminatory HCG zone: its use in the sonographic evaluation for ectopic pregnancy. *Obstet Gynecol* 1981; **58**: 156–161.

Ory SJ, O'Brien PS, Nuadi E, Melton LJ, Hermann R. Fertility after ectopic pregnancy. *Fertil Steril* 1993; **60**: 137–139.

FACTS YOU SHOULD HAVE LEARNT . . .

▶ **The diagnosis and assessment of ectopic pregnancy**
▶ **The discriminatory role of hCG assay**
▶ **The treatment options in ectopic pregnancy**

CASE 6

Recurrent miscarriage

A 27-year-old woman was admitted as an emergency with a history of lower abdominal pain and heavy vaginal bleeding over the previous 24 hours. She had had 7 weeks' amenorrhoea and a positive pregnancy test. On examination, she was in a stable condition but was acutely tender suprapubically. On vaginal examination, the cervix was open with a gestation sac distending it. This was removed with sponge-holding forceps and the bleeding eased a little. A diagnosis of incomplete abortion was made and the patient underwent evacuation of retained products. The presence of retained products was later confirmed histologically.

Before going home, the patient raised concerns that she had previously had two early miscarriages during the past 18 months, both of which required surgical evacuation. She questioned whether there was anything wrong with her reproductive activity.

Q1: How would you counsel her at this stage?

An appointment was made to review the case 6 weeks later and to arrange further investigations.

Q2: Which of the following are possible causes of recurrent miscarriage?
A: Pituitary microadenoma.
B: Polycystic ovarian syndrome.
C: Pelvic kidney.
D: Cervical incompetence.
E: Progesterone deficiency.

At the outpatient consultation, it transpired that all three miscarriages had occurred with the same partner and that he had not been responsible for any other pregnancies. Examination of the woman revealed normal pelvic anatomy. They were counselled about the different causes of recurrent miscarriage and were reassured that it was unlikely that a cause would be found and that a subsequent pregnancy would have a good chance of successful outcome. Arrangements were made to perform a number of blood tests on both partners and to see them with the results 2 months later.

Q3: Which of the following blood tests would you perform?
A: Parental karyotyping.
B: Thyroid function tests.
C: Serial progesterone assays.

D: TORCH screen.

E: Lupus anticoagulant.

The karyotypes were 46XX and 46XY, and all the hormonal assays were normal. There was no expression of antipaternal antibodies or of lupus anticoagulants.

It was suggested that the woman should undergo hysterosalpingography.

Q4:   What is the purpose of a hysterosalpingogram in this context?

The hysterosalpingogram showed a normal cervical canal with a single uterine cavity. However, there were some filling defects within that cavity. These were not suggestive of a septum.

On further questioning, she admitted that whilst her menstrual periods had always been regular since her first miscarriage they had tended to be very painful and lighter than previously.

Q5:   What is the likely diagnosis and how would you proceed?

Hysteroscopic examination of the uterine cavity confirmed adhesions, which were broken down by laser ablation under the same anaesthetic. There were no remaining adhesions at the end of the procedure, with normal uterine anatomy having been restored.

Q6:   How would you manage her now?

She remained on hormone replacement therapy with an intrauterine device (IUD) *in situ* for 3 months, during which time she menstruated regularly. Her periods were still painful and were a little heavier than previously, although this may have been related to the IUD. She was very keen to try for another pregnancy and the IUD was removed.

Six months later, she presented with a positive pregnancy test and an ultrasound scan showed an intrauterine gestation.

Q7:   What are the risks of pregnancy in this case?

COMMENTARY

Immediately following a third miscarriage, a woman is unlikely to be ready for detailed counselling about possible causes. It is important to be as supportive as possible and perhaps the best possible reassurance is that, even though she has had three consecutive miscarriages, the chance of subsequent pregnancies being successful is greater than the chance of a miscarriage occurring. Stirrat (1990) quotes the likelihood of a successful outcome being between 54 and 75% in this situation. You should also inform her that there are possible causes of recurrent miscarriage and that this would be investigated at her follow-up appointment (**Q1**).

There are numerous aetiological factors, of which the main groups are hormonal, immunological, anatomical, chromosomal and due to collagen disorders. Infections have been implicated in the past. However, although various infections may cause a single miscarriage, the evidence for infective causes of recurrent miscarriage is dubious. Pituitary microadenomas, while hormone secreting, are not thought to be implicated, whereas polycystic ovarian syndrome is becoming increasingly recognized as a cause of recurrent miscarriage. Although a pelvic kidney may be associated with a Mullerian fusion defect of the genital tract, it is not a cause of recurrent pregnancy loss *per se*. Cervical incompetence usually causes mid-trimester loss, but there have been suggestions that it may also be responsible for early pregnancy loss (Edmonds, 1988) (**Q2: true = B, D, E; false = A, C**).

It is useful to send products for fetal karyotyping at the time of evacuation in cases of recurrent miscarriage. Similarly, parental karyotyping is important. There is doubt about whether abnormalities of thyroid function cause miscarriage, and similarly with diabetes, except when there is extremely poor control. Serial progesterone assays are not helpful. A TORCH (toxoplasmosis, rubella, cytomegalovirus, herpes) screen would not be indicated. Lupus anticoagulant expression is the most important indicator of collagen disease associated with recurrent miscarriage along with anticardiolipin antibody estimations (**Q3: true = A, E; false = B, C, D**).

In the absence of any identified abnormality with the above investigations, the purpose of hysterosalpingography would be to look for an anatomical cause of miscarriage. Such problems identified by this would be congenital uterine abnormality, intrauterine adhesions (Ashermann's syndrome) and possible cervical incompetence if carried out premenstrually (**Q4**). The presence of filling defects within the endometrial cavity with a history of very painful periods since the first evacuation of the uterus would be highly suggestive of intrauterine adhesions being responsible for the recurrent miscarriages (**Q5**).

With the suspicion of intrauterine adhesions, the correct management is hysteroscopy with an attempt to try to break down the adhesions during the same procedure. There is a risk of the adhesions recurring. To minimize this, you should leave an intrauterine device *in situ* for several months to separate the anterior and posterior uterine walls whilst administering cyclical oestrogen and progestogen therapy to try to stimulate regular endometrial development throughout the uterine cavity (**Q6**).

Should conception occur following treatment of Ashermann's syndrome, there is still a risk of abnormal implantation which may cause miscarriage or premature labour. In addition, there is a significant risk of excessive placental implantation (placenta accreta), making the risk of significant postpartum haemorrhage and even hysterectomy a real possibility (**Q7**).

REFERENCES

Edmonds DE. Use of cervical cerclage in patients with recurrent first trimester abortion. In: Beard RW, Sharp F (eds) *Early Pregnancy Loss*, pp 411–415. London: Springer, 1988.

Stirrat GM. Recurrent miscarriage I and II. *Lancet* 1990; **336**: 673–675 and 724–733.

FACTS YOU SHOULD HAVE LEARNT . . .

▶ The aetiology and investigation of recurrent miscarriage
▶ The diagnosis and management of Ashermann's syndrome
▶ Complications of pregnancy associated with previous Ashermann's syndrome

CASE 7

Microcephaly

A 16-year-old P0+0 woman was admitted to the gynaecology ward at 11 weeks' gestation with vaginal bleeding. She was a smoker and had recently left a children's home to live with a foster mother. On admission, the bleeding had ceased and she was otherwise asymptomatic. General and abdominal examination findings were unremarkable, and on vaginal examination the uterine size was compatible with her gestation and the cervical os was closed. An offensive vaginal discharge was noted and high vaginal and endocervical swabs were taken. An ultrasound scan was unremarkable, with the fetal heart seen. She was discharged home, although when the endocervical swab indicated a chlamydial infection she and her partner were referred to the genitourinary medicine clinic.

When she attended the antenatal booking clinic at 15 weeks' gestation, her history was largely unchanged, although she had another episode of vaginal bleeding 1 week previously which had resolved. Investigations, which included maternal serum screening for neural tube defects and Down's syndrome, were unremarkable. However, when she attended for a detailed ultrasound scan at 20 weeks' gestation, the fetus was reported as microcephalic; the biparietal diameter was 37 mm and the head circumference 144 mm (equivalent to 16 weeks' gestation), the abdominal circumference was 156 mm (equivalent to 20 weeks' gestation) and the femur length was 290 mm (equivalent to 19 weeks' gestation). Echogenic bowel was noted, but no other abnormalities were found.

> **Q1:** What is meant by microcephaly and what is the incidence of the condition?
>
> **Q2:** Which of the following statements concerning microcephaly are correct?
> A: The majority of microcephalic infants have learning impairment.
> B: In general, the smaller the head the worse the prognosis.
> C: Despite microcephaly, a child may have normal intelligence.
> D: Delivery is frequently complicated by shoulder dystocia.
>
> **Q3:** What is the significance of echogenic bowel?
>
> **Q4:** What investigation of the cause of microcephaly would you have instigated?

A TORCH (toxoplasmosis, rubella, cytomegalovirus, herpes) screen was strongly suggestive of a recent cytomegalovirus (CMV) infection. In the view of the ultrasonographic findings, a range of options, including invasive methods of assessing a possible *in utero* infection, and termination of pregnancy were discussed. She did not wish any invasive procedure, as she was not prepared to consider termination of pregnancy under any circumstances.

Q5: **What are the typical symptoms of a maternal CMV infection?**

Q6: **Which of the following statements concerning the spread of CMV are correct?**
A: CMV can be transmitted via blood transfusion.
B: Transplacental passage of CMV may occur in both primary and secondary infection, leading to congenital infection.
C: Transplacental transmission rates in primary infection are approximately 70%.
D: Infants may be infected by the virus excreted in breast milk.
E: The prevalence of CMV infection is highest in developed countries.

Q7: **How could you have confirmed the *in utero* diagnosis of CMV infection?**

The patient received counselling from a paediatrician regarding the possible complications that her baby would face after delivery.

Q8: **Which of the following statements concerning congenital CMV infection are correct?**
A: The incidence of congenital CMV infection is between 1:100 and 1:300.
B: Twenty per cent of congenitally infected infants are symptomatic at birth.
C: The infant mortality rate of babies who are symptomatic at birth is 50%.
D: The characteristic defect on follow-up at between 1 and 2 years of age is sensorineural deafness.
E: Some 80–90% of congenitally infected babies develop normally.

Serial ultrasound scans were performed throughout pregnancy. Measurement of biparietal diameter and head circumference remained below the 5th centile. Initial measurements of abdominal circumference (AC) approximated to the 50th centile; however, at 35 weeks' gestation, the AC had fallen below the 10th centile. Intrauterine growth restriction was confirmed at 38 weeks' gestation, when the AC was below the 5th centile and the maximal diameter of the largest pool of amniotic fluid was 2 cm. At that time the patient also reported a reduction in fetal movements and a decision was taken to induce labour.

After cervical ripening with prostaglandin gel, artificial rupture of membranes and Syntocinon infusion resulted in the delivery of a male infant who weighed 2.36 kg. The labour was not complicated by either fetal distress or shoulder dystocia. Microcephaly was confirmed (head circumference 335 mm) and a widespread petechial rash over the baby's trunk was noted. His liver and spleen were just palpable. He was nursed in a single room (as it was thought likely that he was excreting CMV) and the rash resolved over 6 days. Investigations revealed thrombocytopenia (88×10^9 l^{-1}) and positive CMV titres, and CMV was isolated in a urine sample. The maximal bilirubin level was 141 μmol l^{-1} but no phototherapy was needed. A cranial ultrasound scan showed a generalized increase in echogenicity of the white matter, consistent with CMV infection. He suffered no complications before discharge after 6 days fully breast fed. However, on subsequent paediatric follow-up, brainstem-evoked response audiometry studies indicated a profound sensorineural deafness, and there were early signs of delayed development.

Q9: Do you think congenital CMV infection can be prevented? In particular:
A: Is screening of antenatal patients indicated?
B: Do CMV vaccines exist?
C: Is treatment of maternal CMV infection warranted?

The mother attended for a routine 6-week postnatal review, and the puerperium was uncomplicated. She was keen to know when she could have another child and whether that child would also be affected.

Q10: What would your answer have been?

COMMENTARY

Microcephaly means 'small head', but the clinical importance of the entity is its association with microencephaly ('small brain') and intellectual disability. There is no universally accepted definition, but a head circumference more than three standard deviations below the mean correlates much better with learning impairment than a head circumference more than two standard deviations below the mean. The incidence of the former is approximately 1:7000 (**Q1**).

It is difficult to make definitive statements concerning the prognosis of an entity such as microcephaly with an unclear definition and multiple aetiologies. Extreme caution should be used when counselling couples when an *in utero* diagnosis of microcephaly is made. Several general remarks are, however, appropriate: most microcephalic infants have difficulties learning (many severely), and the prognosis tends to worsen the smaller the fetal head is. If microcephaly is part of a genetic syndrome (e.g. Meckel's syndrome), the outcome is uniformly poor. Uncomplicated delivery is anticipated in cases of microcephaly, although shoulder dystocia occasionally occurs due to incomplete dilatation of the cervix by the small head (**Q2: true = A, B, C; false = D**).

Although echogenic areas of bowel (which appear as bright reflections with shadowing on ultrasound scans) are usually a normal variant, they may represent features of cystic fibrosis, CMV infection and several chromosomal abnormalities (**Q3**).

The search for the cause of microcephaly must include a careful history; in particular, any relevant family history, or any history suggestive of teratogen exposure, alcohol abuse or maternal infection, must be sought. Because microcephaly is part of many malformation syndromes, a careful search using ultrasonography for any other associated anomalies is warranted. Microcephaly is part of the clinical TORCH syndrome (toxoplasmosis, rubella, cytomegalovirus, herpes) and maternal blood should be sent for a TORCH screen. Invasive techniques to karyotype the fetus (amniocentesis or chorionic villus biopsy) should also be considered. The possibility of performing cordocentesis to measure immunoglobulin (Ig) M in fetal serum after 20 weeks' gestation provides a further option (**Q4**).

Both primary and secondary CMV infections in immunocompetent hosts are usually asymptomatic. Occasionally primary infection may give rise to an infectious mononucleosis syndrome, with a syndrome of fever, atypical lymphocytosis, some malaise, mild lymphadenopathy, but generally has a benign course. This manifestation of CMV infection is usually self-limiting, although the fever may last more than 1 month in a few cases. Rarely, serious complications of the acute infection can occur, including interstitial pneumonitis, hepatitis, myocarditis and thrombocytopenia (**Q5**).

Although CMV infection is usually acquired via perinatal transmission and sexual transmission, it may be transmitted via transfused blood and bone marrow. Transplacental passage of CMV may occur in both primary and secondary infection, leading to congenital infection. Transplacental transmission rates in primary maternal infection are approximately 30–40%. Early in life, the infant may be infected transplacentally, by exposure to virus from the cervix at birth, and from the virus excreted in breast milk. Another source of childhood infection is exposure to other babies in nurseries, as infected children shed the virus in urine and in respiratory tract secretions, for much longer than infected adults. The prevalence of CMV infection is higher in underdeveloped countries and in lower socioeconomic populations. It is apparent that sexual activity (higher number of partners, and lower age at onset of sexual activity) correlates with CMV isolation from the cervix (**Q6: true = A, B, D; false = C, E**).

Diagnosis of *in utero* CMV infection may be accomplished in a number of ways. Ultrasonographic demonstration of significant fetal abnormalities (as in this case) provides strongly supportive evidence. The virus may be isolated in fluid collected at amniocentesis, and fetal blood sampling (by cordocentesis) may enable the demonstration of serological, viral or haematological evidence of CMV. Pathological examination of the products of conception after miscarriage or therapeutic abortion may reveal histological evidence of CMV-associated viral changes. After delivery, diagnosis is by isolation of IgM anti-CMV antibodies in cord blood, or by the isolation of CMV from a neonatal urine sample in the first 3 weeks of life (**Q7**).

Congenital CMV infection is the commonest congenital infection in the UK, with an incidence of between 1:100 and 1:300. Some 5–10% of babies congenitally infected with CMV are symptomatic at birth (cytomegalic inclusion disease). This equates to 200 or 300 severely damaged CMV-infected babies in the UK each year. The signs of cytomegalic inclusion disease at birth are those of the classical TORCH syndrome and include microcephaly, hepatosplenomegaly, petechiae, thrombocytopenia and hyperbilirubinaemia. On follow-up, there is a 20% infant mortality rate, and survivors have significant morbidity which can be severe, for example learning disability, spastic diplegia, blindness and deafness. Of the infected neonates delivered without demonstrable disease, 5–15% are at risk of developing some abnormality attributable to CMV before their second birthday, primarily sensorineural hearing loss (**Q8: true = A, D, E; false = B, C**).

Strategies for the prevention of congenital CMV infection are controversial. CMV infections are asymptomatic, thus susceptibility to, and diagnosis of, infection have to be determined by serological screening. The current position in the UK is that screening all antenatal sera for the presence of anti-CMV antibodies is not indicated because serious congenital infection can arise from both seronegative and seropositive women at any stage in pregnancy (Editorial, 1989). In addition, avoidance of CMV infection by seronegative women is not practical (**Q9A**). Prevention of infection in the mother is an attractive strategy. However, although the development of a specific CMV vaccine to effect active immunization against the virus is the subject of intense research efforts, no such vaccine exists. Passive immunization with specific anti-CMV immunoglobulin appears to be useful only as prophylaxis in cases of renal and marrow transplantation (**Q9B**). There is no accepted therapy for acute maternal or neonatal infection, although future avenues for research include prenatal use of antiviral drugs to prevent or modify intrauterine infection (**Q9C**).

Advice regarding future pregnancies after a child has suffered from congenital CMV infection is difficult; the patient could not be given the reassurance that she was seeking. Viral shedding can continue for extended periods of time, and no data are available to extrapolate a safe waiting interval. Although severe transplacental infection is not usually seen in children of women with pre-existing antibody, subsequent pregnancies in women with one affected infant have resulted in mildly infected neonates (**Q10**).

REFERENCE

Editorial. Screening for congenital CMV. *Lancet* 1989; **ii**: 599–600.

FACTS YOU SHOULD HAVE LEARNT . . .

▶ **The importance and investigation of microcephaly**
▶ **The fetal and maternal risks of cytomegalovirus**
▶ **The management options in pregnancies complicated by cytomegalovirus infection**

CASE 8

Abdominal pain

A 27-year-old P1 + 1 woman at 32 weeks' gestation was admitted to the hospital antenatal ward after initially presenting to her general practitioner with a 4-hour history of central backache, abdominal pain (constant with exacerbations), nausea and vomiting. She denied any history of bowel symptoms, but had noted some slight urinary frequency. There was no relevant past medical history; her previous child had been delivered normally after an uncomplicated pregnancy, 4 years previously. She denied any alcohol ingestion in pregnancy.

On examination, she was found to be hyperventilating and was distressed with pain. She was apyrexial, her pulse was 94 beats per minute, and her blood pressure was 110/60 mmHg. Her abdomen was soft, with mild epigastric and right loin tenderness. There was no rebound tenderness or guarding. The uterus was soft and non-tender, and the fetal heart was heard. Urinalysis revealed a proteinuria 1+ with no haematuria.

A provisional diagnosis of pyelonephritis was made. Intravenous antibiotic therapy was commenced and a 150-mg pethidine injection was administered intramuscularly. A urine specimen was sent for urgent microscopy.

QI: **What microorganisms are commonly responsible for urinary tract infections in pregnancy?**

Q2: **Which of the following intravenous therapies could be prescribed safely?**
A: Ciprofloxacin.
B: Nitrofurantoin.
C: Ampicillin.
D: Cefoxitin.
E: Gentamicin.

The haemoglobin was 12.1 $g\,dl^{-1}$, the white cell count was $21 \times 10^9\,l^{-1}$ (neutrophils $18.3 \times 10^9\,l^{-1}$), and platelet count was $381 \times 10^9\,l^{-1}$. Urgent urinary microscopy was unremarkable, and subsequent cultures were negative.

Over the 4 hours following admission there was a marked increase in the intensity of the abdominal pain, especially in the right upper quadrant. On examination there was rebound tenderness and guarding over this area, with hypoactive bowel sounds. The amylase level was checked and found to be $238\ U\,l^{-1}$ (normal $40–120\ U\,l^{-1}$); urea and electrolytes, liver function tests, and glucose levels were all within the normal range.

Q3: Which of the following should be included in the differential diagnosis?
A: HELLP syndrome.
B: Appendicitis.
C: Cholecystitis.
D: Acute fatty liver of pregnancy.
E: Pancreatitis.

Q4: What investigation would you instigate, and why?

Some 12 hours following admission, the patient's condition had deteriorated further and a general surgical opinion was sought. She was complaining of increased abdominal pain and was pyrexial (37.9°C). There was increased tenderness and guarding in the right upper quadrant on abdominal examination. A repeat white cell count was 19×10^9 l^{-1} (neutrophils 17.1×10^9 l^{-1}). An ultrasound scan revealed no abnormality in the biliary tract, liver, pancreas, spleen or left kidney. There was mild dilatation of the right pelvicalyceal system which was thought to be consistent with pregnancy. A single live fetus was noted with abdominal and head circumference measurements within the normal range. No abruption was seen. The decision was made to perform a laparotomy in a further 12 hours if her clinical condition had not improved.

Q5: Would you have recommended that a laparotomy be performed earlier? Why?

Q6: Concerning the differential diagnosis of appendicitis in pregnancy: which of the following statements are correct?
A: The incidence of appendicitis in pregnant women is lower than that in non-pregnant women.
B: The finding of pain in the right *upper* quadrant made the diagnosis less likely.
C: Unless perforation has occurred, maternal and perinatal mortality rates are very low.
D: The raised serum amylase level excluded the diagnosis.
E: Conservative management is optimal, to avoid the dangers of anaesthesia.

After a further 12 hours, her condition was largely unchanged. She still complained of severe right-sided abdominal pain and remained pyrexial (37.8°C). A laparotomy was performed.

Q7: What incision would you recommend?

At laparotomy, an oedematous mass in head of pancreas was noted. The appendix, liver, gallbladder, stomach, small intestine and colon were found to be normal. An excess of serous peritoneal free fluid was noted (samples were sent to microbiology and virology laboratories for culture). A diagnosis of pancreatitis in pregnancy was made.

Q8: Does pregnancy predispose to pancreatitis?

Q9: Concerning the diagnosis of pancreatitis in pregnancy, which of the following statements are correct?
A: The optimal diagnostic test would have been emergency endoscopic retrograde cholangiopancreatography.
B: Most cases eventually require emergency surgery.
C: The incidence is lower than appendicitis in pregnancy.
D: It most frequently occurs in the third trimester of pregnancy.
E: Drug ingestion is a common cause.

Q10: What additional investigations should you arrange?

Q11: When you are considering her postoperative management:
A: Oral intake should be strongly encouraged.
B: Serum amylase levels should fall within 72 hours.
C: Parenteral narcotics are contraindicated.
D: Tocolytic therapy is of proven benefit.

The postoperative recovery was largely uncomplicated, as was the remainder of her pregnancy which culminated in the normal delivery of a female infant of 3.28 kg at 39 weeks' gestation. Additional investigations, including culture of the peritoneal fluid and serial viral serology, were unremarkable, and the aetiology of the pancreatitis remained unclear.

COMMENTARY

The microorganisms generally responsible for pyelonephritis in pregnancy are *Escherichia coli*, *Klebsiella*, *Enterobacter* and *Proteus* species (**Q1**).

The initial choice of antimicrobial agent in this situation is empiric. Antibacterial agents are among the most commonly used medications in pregnancy, and most are safe drugs in pregnancy. All penicillins are apparently safe in patients not allergic to these drugs. All cephalosporins cross the placenta to a similar degree. Second- and third-generation cephalosporins containing the *N*-methylthiotetrazole side chain have been reported to be associated with testicular hypoplasia in newborn animals, but this has not been seen in humans. Cefoxitin does not contain this side chain and would thus seem to be a rational choice in pregnancy. All the aminoglycosides cross the placenta to some degree, and are associated with a risk of fetal ototoxicity of about 2%. There are no reports of adverse effects following the use of nitrofurantoin in pregnancy although not available for intravenous use (Gilstrap *et al*, 1991). The fluoroquinolones (ciprofloxacin and norfloxacin) are relatively new antibiotics frequently used to treat non-pregnant patients with urinary tract infections. There have been reports of irreversible arthropathy in newborn animals after administration in pregnancy (Gilstrap *et al*, 1991), and it is recommended that these drugs are not prescribed in pregnancy (**Q2: true = C, D; false = A, E; B is not available intravenously**).

Pre-eclampsia with haemolysis, elevated liver enzymes and low platelet count (HELLP syndrome) often presents with severe epigastric or right upper quadrant pain. However, in this case the blood pressure was not raised and liver function and platelet counts were normal. Abdominal pain, nausea and vomiting are common to appendicitis, cholecystitis and pancreatitis, and the clinical findings would not exclude any of these diagnoses. Acute fatty liver of pregnancy presents with vomiting in the third trimester, but is accompanied by a systemic illness manifest as malaise and lethargy for days or weeks followed by jaundice with drowsiness or confusion. In addition, levels of liver enzymes are moderately raised (**Q3: true = B, C, E; false = A, D**).

If the abdominal pain results from cholecystitis, ultrasonographic examination of the gallbladder and common duct reliably demonstrates gallstones and can detect common duct dilatation. Once the diagnosis has been made, conservative treatment with analgesics, intravenous fluids and nasogastric suction should be initiated. Ultrasonography will reveal gallstones in over 50% of cases of pancreatitis, but medical management of pancreatitis and cholecystitis is similar. Ultrasonography contributes little to the diagnosis of appendicitis other than to exclude other conditions such as a degenerating fibroid, ruptured adnexal cyst, ureteric obstruction and placental abruption (**Q4**).

The differential diagnosis clearly included acute appendicitis, the most common surgical condition to accompany pregnancy (1 in 2000 pregnancies). The incidence in pregnant women is the same as that in non-pregnant women (Tamir *et al*, 1990). The maternal risks of peritonitis and sepsis, and the fetal risks of premature labour and fetal demise, are greatest in cases of perforation. When perforation has occurred, maternal and fetal mortality rates of 17% and 43% have been reported, whereas in the absence of perforation these rates are virtually zero (Horowitz *et al*, 1985). The greatest risk in appendicitis in pregnancy is that delays in diagnosis and definitive surgery lead to perforation, and it could be argued that the laparotomy should have been expedited. However, the diagnosis is notoriously difficult. The distortion of abdominal anatomy by the gravid uterus generally leads to displacement of the appendix upwards and to the right with advancing gestation, but many remain in the right lower quadrant or in the vicinity of the kidney, hence the location of maximal pain and tenderness is very variable. Other symptoms of appendicitis may be less evident in pregnancy; normal pregnant women may have a mild leucocytosis, and the raised serum amylase level could be consistent with intraperitoneal inflammation. For these reasons, it is often necessary to observe patients over a number of hours, obtain serial white cell counts and repeat the clinical examination (**Q5 and Q6: true = C; false = A, B, D, E**).

In late pregnancy, the gravid uterus prevents easy access to organs other than the anterior lower segment. Midline or paramedian incisions allow better access than low transverse or McBurney incisions, and can be easily extended if necessary. In this case a right paramedian incision over the area of maximal tenderness was probably optimal (**Q7**).

Pancreatitis in pregnancy is uncommon (between 1:4000 and 1:11 000 pregnancies). Although an association between pregnancy and pancreatitis has been suggested, there are few data to support this theory. Predisposing factors include gallstones (the most common underlying factor in pregnancy), familial hyperlipidaemia, hyperparathyroidism and drug ingestion. The normal increase in lipid levels in the third trimester may explain the predilection of pancreatitis in the third trimester of pregnancy. The drugs most cc nmonly associated with pancreatitis (tetracyclines and thiazide diuretics) are rarely prescribed in pregnancy, thus drug ingestion is an uncommon predisposing factor. In pregnancy, endoscopic cholangiopancreatography and stone extraction is not acceptable owing to heavy radiation exposure of the fetus during screening. Most cases of pancreatitis in pregnancy resolve with conservative management; in one series emergency surgery was necessary in less than 10% of cases (Block and Kelly, 1989) (**Q8 and Q9: true = C, D; false = A, B, E**). Additional investigations should include serum lipids (levels raised in hyperlipidaemia), serum calcium (increased in hyperparathyroidism) and viral titres (which should be repeated after recovery) (**Q10**).

Once a diagnosis of pancreatitis has been made, management consists of supportive care, with careful attention to intravenous fluid replacement with close monitoring of electrolyte, calcium and glucose concentrations. Parenteral narcotics should be administered for pain control, with relatively high doses often required. The patient should not ingest any solids or liquids until all pain has subsided. Although data to support the value of nasogastric suction are unavailable, the procedure is often used. The serum amylase level will usually return to normal with 72 hours of supportive care. Although intravenous tocolytic therapy has not been proven to be of benefit, many advocate tocolysis during the first few days after surgery when the risk of premature labour is greatest (**Q11: true = B; false = A, C, D**).

REFERENCES

Block P, Kelly TR. Management of gallstone pancreatitis during pregnancy and the postpartum period. *Surg Gynecol Obstet* 1989; **168**: 426–428.

Gilstrap LC, Little BB, Cunningham FG. Medication use during pregnancy. Part 2. Special considerations. In: *Williams' Obstetrics*, 18th edn. Norwalk, CT: Appleton & Lange, 1991: Supplement 11.

Horowitz MD, Gomez GA, Santiesbastian R, Burkitt G. Acute appendicitis during pregnancy. *Arch Surg* 1985; **120**: 1362–1367.

Tamir IL, Bongard FS, Klein SR. Acute appendicitis in pregnancy. *Am J Surg* 1990; **160**: 571.

FACTS YOU SHOULD HAVE LEARNT . . .

▶ The microorganisms commonly responsible for pyelonephritis in pregnancy
▶ The differential diagnosis of right upper quadrant abdominal pain in pregnancy
▶ The management of abdominal pain in pregnancy
▶ How to diagnose and manage pancreatitis in pregnancy

CASE 9

Drug addiction

A 16-year-old P0 girl attended the antenatal clinic at 6 weeks' gestation, having been referred by the local drug dependency unit, where she was an inpatient. She gave a 2-year history of having smoked Crack cocaine and she had also been injecting heroin intravenously. She had been working as a prostitute to support her drug habit. She normally lived with foster parents. Her boyfriend (who was also her pimp) had a long history of sexually transmitted diseases (including gonorrhoea) and the patient had recently been treated in the genitourinary medicine clinic for a chlamydial infection.

> **Q1:** **Which of the following statements regarding opiates and cocaine are correct?**
> A: Heroin and cocaine both cross the placenta.
> B: Cocaine can be absorbed across any mucosal surface.
> C: Heroin is derived naturally from opium.
> D: Cocaine is present in blood or urine for up to 6 days after intake.

The patient was worried about the effects that her drug abuse might have had on the baby, but was adamant that she did not want a termination. She wanted to know the risks consequent upon the cocaine and heroin intake.

> **Q2:** **Which of the following conditions are associated with cocaine abuse ?**
> A: Gestational diabetes.
> B: Microcephaly.
> C: A teratogenic effect.
> D: Placental abruption.
> E: Preterm labour.

> **Q3:** **Which of the following conditions are associated with heroin abuse?**
> A: Intrauterine growth restriction.
> B: A teratogenic effect.
> C: Pre-eclampsia.
> D: Preterm labour.
> E: Cardiac arrhythmias

In addition to routine antenatal screening tests, vaginal and cervical swabs were sent for Chlamydia and gonorrhoea culture. Following detailed counselling blood was taken for human immunodeficiency virus (HIV) and hepatitis B status. The results of these investigations, and of syphilis serology, were negative. After discussion with her psychiatrist at the drug dependency unit, it was decided to alter her drug dependence to methadone. She appeared very anxious to comply with 'whatever was best for the baby'.

Q4:   What are the advantages of methadone therapy?

A detailed ultrasound scan was performed at 18 weeks' gestation; no abnormality was seen. At this time the patient had reduced her dependence on methadone to 20 mg per day (from an initial stabilization dose of 30 mg daily). The reduction had involved little discomfort. She said that she had not used any other drug apart from an occasional 10-mg tablet of either diazepam or temazepam. Serial monthly ultrasound scans were planned.

Unfortunately, she left the drug dependency unit at 20 weeks' gestation and travelled to London with her boyfriend. She returned alone at 30 weeks' gestation, and asked her foster parents if she could rejoin them. She stated that she had been forced to leave by her boyfriend, and expressed relief at having returned. She gave a history of further heroin and cocaine abuse and of prostitution. She also claimed to have been admitted to hospital with a heroin overdose but was unable to provide further details.

Q5:   What are the signs of heroin overdose?

Q6:   What is the treatment for acute heroin overdose?

An ultrasound scan was performed at 31 weeks' gestation; good fetal growth and normal liquor volume were noted. The patient restarted the methadone programme. A case conference was held, and after some debate it was decided that, after delivery, she and her baby should live with her foster parents (at least in the short term). An ultrasound scan at 35 weeks' gestation was unremarkable, at this time she had reduced her methadone intake to 15 mg per day. She remained asymptomatic until she was admitted in spontaneous labour at 38 weeks' gestation.

Q7:   What would be your management plan for her labour?

After an uncomplicated labour, a female infant weighing 3.06 kg was delivered in good condition.

Q8:   Which of the following statements regarding the puerperium are correct?
A: If neonatal withdrawal syndrome occurs, it will be apparent by 5 days following delivery.

B: If a mother is addicted to heroin, breastfeeding is contraindicated.

C: If a mother is addicted to methadone, breastfeeding is contraindicated.

D: If a drug addict wishes to breastfeed, HIV status should be checked.

Her baby daughter developed irritability and sneezing on day 1, and became very agitated with vomiting at 42 hours post-delivery. The baby was treated with oral morphine and underwent a gradual reduction in dose over the next 10 days. She was irritable and inconsolable at various stages during the withdrawal, but was receiving no treatment for 4 days before discharge at 16 days post-delivery. The baby was initially breastfed, but on discharge was fully bottle-fed. Her mother's puerperium was wholly uncomplicated.

COMMENTARY

Both heroin and cocaine abuse have increased in recent years. Natural opiates, such as codeine and morphine, are obtained from the opium-producing poppy. Heroin and methadone are synthetic derivatives of opium. Heroin is the drug of choice amongst addicts, probably because it has a rapid action. Cocaine is derived from a coca plant, and is available in a water-soluble form which can be absorbed from any mucosal surface (hence 'snorting'). Cocaine is a drug of abuse because it produces euphoria and mental stimulation. It is present in blood or urine for only about 12 hours after intake, although stable metabolites can be found for up to 6 days. Both drugs freely cross the placenta (**Q1: true = A, B; false = C, D**).

Assessment of the risks of drugs of abuse are compounded by socioeconomic and environmental factors. Cocaine has been identified as a teratogenic agent, and a variety of abnormalities have been reported. Vasospasm of both fetal and maternal circulations appears to be the responsible mechanism. Cerebral infarction may result in motor or intellectual impairment. The most commonly measurable fetal abnormality is microcephaly. The vasospasm and hypertension caused by cocaine (secondary to increased catecholamine concentrations) result in the increased incidence of placental abruption. Other adverse effects of cocaine intake in pregnancy include preterm labour, premature rupture of membranes, intrauterine growth restriction and an increased incidence of stillbirth (**Q2: true = B, C, D, E; false = A**). Heroin does not seem to be associated with an increased risk of teratogenicity, although contaminants of drugs sold on the street, such as strychnine, may be teratogenic. Heroin is, however, clearly associated with intrauterine growth restriction and preterm labour. It is cocaine intake that can cause cardiac arrhythmias (**Q3: true = A, D; false = B, C, E**).

The advantage of methadone is that it can be taken orally, is long acting and constant blood levels are achieved. In addition, by prescribing the drug in a controlled fashion, it is hoped that the problems associated with street drug use and the accompanying high-risk sexual behaviour are reduced. Methadone is the only drug available to treat opioid-addicted women. The easiest way to determine the optimal dose of methadone (to avoid both intoxication and withdrawal symptoms) is to admit a pregnant addict to a drug dependency unit. The aim is to achieve the lowest acceptable dose without cravings. If a dose below 20 mg per day can be attained, only a minority of babies will develop signs of withdrawal. There is some debate as to whether methadone maintenance or detoxification programmes are the best form of treatment. If detoxification is attempted, the dose should be reduced at 2–5 mg per week, with most of the reduction in the second trimester (**Q4**).

An acute heroin overdose is life threatening to both mother and baby. It results in varying degrees of unresponsiveness, hypothermia, respiratory depression and bradycardia. If advanced, the pupils dilate, and the skin becomes cyanotic as the circulation fails (**Q5**). If the patient is unresponsive, an endotracheal tube should be inserted. The administration of the antagonist naloxone is both therapeutic and diagnostic. An intravenous dose of 0.5–1 mg can be given on more than one occasion, at 5-minute intervals, until respiration improves. After stabilization, sneezing, pruritus and urinary retention are common problems (**Q6**).

In labour, the normal daily methadone maintenance dose should be given. Opiate analgesia is not contraindicated, but larger doses than normal will be necessary. Narcotics with significant agonist–antagonist properties, such as pentazocine, should not be given, for fear of precipitating a withdrawal syndrome (**Q7**).

Signs of neonatal withdrawal syndrome include shaking, sweating, seizures, sneezing, pyrexia, diarrhoea and vomiting. If a mother is taking heroin, these signs are usually apparent within 3–5 days of delivery. The half-life of methadone is longer, thus the babies may present with signs of withdrawal up to 2 weeks after delivery if mothers have taken methadone. If a mother remains addicted to heroin, breastfeeding is contraindicated. However, if the methadone intake of an addict is less than 20 mg per day (as in this case), breastfeeding is probably not contraindicated – and may reduce the severity of neonatal withdrawal syndrome. There is a significant risk of HIV transmission via breast milk; thus if a drug addict wishes to breastfeed, it is appropriate to check HIV status (**Q8: true = B, D; false = A, C**).

FACTS YOU SHOULD HAVE LEARNT . . .

▶ **The risks of drug addiction in pregnancy**
▶ **The management of drug addiction in pregnancy, especially methadone therapy**
▶ **The management of drug addicts and their babies in the puerperium**

CASE 10

Endocrine disease

A 31-year-old P1 + 1 Caucasian married woman was referred to the fertility clinic 18 months after a right salpingectomy for a tubal ectopic pregnancy.

Q1:   Which of the following statements are correct?
A: The World Health Organization definition of subfertility would consider this situation as secondary infertility.
B: The most likely cause for the delay in conception is tubal disease.
C: Tubal disease is the commonest cause of secondary subfertility.
D: All tubal pregnancies are a consequence of pelvic inflammatory disease.
E: This woman has a 10% chance of delivering a term baby in the future.

The patient had one child; a 2.86-kg male was delivered normally at 37 weeks' gestation following spontaneous conception. She suffered from insulin-dependent diabetes and myxoedema (for the latter she took 100 µg thyroxine daily). She had been diagnosed with insulin-dependent diabetes at the age of 12 years and her control was thought to be good on a twice-daily regimen of soluble (12 units) and isophane (12 units) insulin.

Q2:   What would be your advice if you were consulted by this patient?
A: To advise sterilization as she has serious maternal disease.
B: To advise against pregnancy due to maternal ingestion of thyroxine.
C: To advise her to commence ingestion of 400 mg folic acid daily.
D: To advise her to avoid pregnancy and to use the progestogen-only contraceptive pill.
E: To advise her to optimize her diabetic control.

On examination, the patient had a background retinopathy but there was no evidence of diabetic nephropathy or neuropathy. She was a non-smoker and her menstrual pattern was regular, lasting 4 days every month. Her last menstrual period was 6 weeks previously. There was no overt history of any pelvic inflammatory disease and the pelvis was noted to have been normal at the time of laparotomy.

A pregnancy test was positive.

Q3:   How would you manage the early stages of this pregnancy?

When seen at a subsequent consultation she had experienced 8 weeks' amenorrhoea and an ultrasound scan confirmed a singleton viable intrauterine pregnancy with a crown–rump length of 18 mm, consistent with the gestational age. The blood pressure was 110/70 mmHg.

Q4: **Which of the following statements concerning insulin-dependent diabetes and pregnancy are correct?**
A: There is an increased risk of Down's syndrome.
B: Maternal serum screening for Down's syndrome is invalid.
C: The incidence of neural tube defects is increased.
D: Optimizing pre-conception glucose levels can significantly reduce the risk of structural fetal abnormalities.
E: There is an increased risk of spontaneous miscarriage.

Q5: **How would you manage her antenatal care?**

Q6: **Which of the following statements about pregnant insulin-dependent diabetics are correct (compared with the general pregnant population)?**
A: They have a greater risk of developing pre-eclampsia.
B: They have a greater risk of preterm delivery.
C: They have no greater risk of post-Caesarean section febrile morbidity.
D: They have no greater risk of shoulder dystocia.
E: They have a greater risk of going blind.

The patient was seen in the joint antenatal/diabetes clinic at 11 weeks' gestation. The blood pressure was 110/70 mmHg and the body mass index was 26 (kg m^{-2}). Dipstick testing of urine revealed 2+ glucose and no proteinuria. The serum fructosamine level was 1.9 μmol l^{-1}, the free thyroxine concentration was 11.7 pmol l^{-1} and the level of thyroid stimulating hormone (TSH) was 2.3 mU l^{-1}. The insulin regimen was changed to a three times a day post-prandial soluble insulin (10 units) with the addition of isophane insulin (16 units) with the evening dose.

At 21 weeks' gestation the free thyroxine concentration was 10.0 pmol l^{-1} and the TSH level was 4.3 mU l^{-1}. Thyroxine replacement therapy was thus increased to 150 μg daily. The retinopathy remained unchanged.

Q7: **What are the complications of aiming for good blood sugar control?**

The pregnancy progressed satisfactorily until 32 weeks' gestation when the patient was admitted to hospital with hypertension (160/90 mmHg) and 2+ proteinuria. Thyroid function test results had remained within the normal range.

The blood pressure remained raised, urine culture was negative and significant proteinuria was confirmed (1.1 g per 24 hours). The haemoglobin concentration was 12.1 g dl^{-1} and the platelet count was 141 $\times$ 10^9 l^{-1}. A diagnosis of pre-eclampsia was made and the decision to deliver the baby was taken. Dexamethasone 12 mg intramuscularly was administered after an insulin infusion had commenced and the dose was repeated 12 hours later. The paediatricians were notified of the impending delivery.

Q8: How would you decide the mode of delivery in this case?

On vaginal examination, the Bishop's score was seven, and a decision to aim for a vaginal delivery was made. Labour was induced by an artificial rupture of the membranes and a Syntocinon infusion was commenced.

Q9: How would you manage the labour?

An epidural catheter was sited and used, and 4 hours later a baby girl was delivered in good condition with a birthweight of 2.1 kg. The baby had an uncomplicated neonatal period and was discharged from the neonatal unit at 21 days of age.

The puerperium was uncomplicated and the patient's blood pressure settled quickly to pre-pregnancy levels. At the 6-week postnatal visit, urinalysis was negative and her blood pressure was 110/70 mmHg.

Q10: What would you advise this woman about thyroxine ingestion during the puerperium?

The thyroid function tests revealed a free thyroxine concentration of 15.2 pmol l^{-1} and the TSH level was 0.1 mU l^{-1}. The baby was thriving and was bottle-fed. The mother was using the progestogen-only pill and requested sterilization.

COMMENTARY

The World Health Organization considers 2 years of unprotected sexual intercourse as part of their definition of subfertility. The reason for this is that 50% of couples who have not conceived after 1 year will conceive in the second year with no intervention. Tubal disease is the commonest cause of secondary subfertility as ascending infection after pregnancy is common. Approximately one third of women who have had an ectopic pregnancy will have another child, although this low proportion may be partly due to women deciding not to have another pregnancy after an ectopic pregnancy (**Q1: true = B, C; false = A, D, E**).

This woman presented with serious endocrine disorders but there is no need to advise against a second pregnancy if the local resources will allow adequate advice and monitoring of the pregnancy. Maternal ingestion of thyroxine is associated with an increased risk of hypoxic ischaemic encephalopathy, cerebral palsy and congenital thyrotoxicosis in the child (Adamson *et al*, 1995) but that does not necessitate a recommendation for sterilization. The presence of thyroid microsomal antibodies (more recently described as thyroid peroxidase antibody, TPO-Ab) in the maternal circulation is strongly associated with postpartum thyroid dysfunction which is, in turn, associated with postpartum depressive illness and is possibly a marker of impaired child development (Pop *et al*, 1995). Folic acid daily is recommended for all woman at a dose of 400 *micrograms* per day before conception and up to 12 weeks' gestation. Folic acid 5 mg daily is recommended for women with previous neural tube defects. Although there is no specific evidence that this will reduce the chances of neural tube defects in other high-risk situations such as diabetes and epilepsy, it would seem to be a reasonable and safe recommendation. The progestogen-only oral contraceptive pill is contraindicated in a woman with a previous ectopic pregnancy; moreover, the combined pill is not contraindicated in diabetes (**Q2: true = E; false = A, B, C, D**).

The management of the early stages of this pregnancy centred around the exclusion of an ectopic gestation, and this should be excluded by an early ultrasound scan to confirm an intrauterine pregnancy (**Q3**).

Pregnant women with insulin-dependent diabetes do not have an increased risk of Down's syndrome. Maternal serum screening for Down's syndrome is invalid due to lower levels of α-fetoprotein observed in diabetic pregnancies. However, there is a greater risk of neural tube defects. Optimizing pre-conception glucose levels can significantly reduce the risk of structural fetal abnormalities. However, these women are more prone to spontaneous miscarriage, especially those with diabetes of long duration and established small vessel disease (**Q4: true = B, C, D, E; false = A**).

Perinatal and maternal mortality have declined appreciably since diabetic pregnancies have been managed in dedicated antenatal clinics with a consultant diabetologist, diabetic nurse, dietician and consultant obstetrician. The aim is to keep fasting blood glucose values below 5.0 mmol l^{-1} and post-prandial (90 minutes) values below 7.0 mmol l^{-1} throughout pregnancy. Anomaly scans should exclude any structural abnormalities and regular growth scans will identify fetal 'overgrowth' and the risk of fetal macrosomia. Problems with blood sugar control may require admission and monitoring, and complications such as urinary infections and pre-eclampsia have to be diagnosed early (**Q5**).

Pregnant women with insulin-dependent diabetes are at greater risk of developing pre-eclampsia and of preterm delivery compared with the general population. They are also at greater risk of post-Caesarean section febrile morbidity and uterine infection, and antibiotic prophylaxis is of proven benefit. Shoulder dystocia is much more common in macrosomic babies and is a real cause for concern. This needs to be considered when assessing the mode of delivery and elective Caesarean section should be performed if the estimated fetal weight is greater than 4.5 kg. Diabetics with proliferative retinopathy need input from a consultant ophthalmologist and all pregnant women with diabetes should have their optic fundi monitored at least three times during the pregnancy. Severe retinopathy should be a contraindication to pregnancy but, if well managed, the risk of retinal haemorrhage can be minimized (**Q6: true = A, B, E; false = C, D**).

The main complication of optimizing control of blood sugar levels is the risk of hypoglycaemic attacks, especially at night. Some women develop a great fear of hypoglycaemia and prefer to accept higher blood sugar levels to avoid this complication. Nocturnal hypoglycaemia causes a rebound hyperglycaemia by the morning, leading to high pre-breakfast levels, which in turn cause loss of control throughout the rest of the day (**Q7**).

When discussing any management decision, you need to be able to demonstrate clinical maturity by discussing the possible options and justifying your choice. Your decision would depend on the previous labour, the presenting part and the physical nature of the cervix, the well-being of the mother and fetus and the availability of adequate monitoring in labour for both the mother and baby. Elective Caesarean section will have risks for the mother (related to the operation, the anaesthetic, thrombosis, infection and postnatal depression) and the baby (an increased likelihood of hyaline membrane lung disease). However, a Caesarean section may be beneficial to prevent intrapartum fetal acidosis especially in the presence of pre-eclampsia. Moreover, if the pre-eclamptic process was severe and difficult to control, then Caesarean section may be safer for the mother. (The management of pre-eclampsia is discussed further in case 20.) This woman's parity was a factor in favour of vaginal delivery (**Q8**).

Management of labour should include an insulin infusion with a sliding scale to maintain euglycaemia, supplemented with a 5% or 10% dextrose infusion. Your aim should be to induce labour and hope for a successful induction of labour and good progress in labour. Any delay or problems should result in early recourse to Caesarean section. Epidural analgesia is to be recommended to maintain metabolic homoeostasis. No problems with the second stage would be anticipated because the labour is preterm. The fetus should be monitored throughout (**Q9**).

This woman's thyroxine ingestion should remain the same for at least 4 weeks and thyroid function tests should be repeated with consideration given to reducing the dose of thyroxine to the pre-pregnancy dose (100 µg) at the 6 weeks' postpartum visit. Usually you should expect to reduce the dose of thyroxine following the fall in the oestrogen-induced production of thyroid binding globulin by the liver that is observed in pregnancy (**Q10**).

REFERENCES

Adamson SJ, Alessandri LM, Badawi N, Burton PR, Pemberton PJ, Stanley F. Predictors of neonatal encephalopathy in full term infants. *BMJ* 1995; **311**: 598–602.

Pop VJ, De Vries E, Van Baar A *et al.* Maternal thyroid peroxidase antibodies during pregnancy: a marker of impaired child development. *J Clin Endocrinol Metab* 1995; **80**: 3561–3566.

FACTS YOU SHOULD HAVE LEARNT . . .

- The prognosis after an ectopic pregnancy
- The complications and management of diabetes in pregnancy
- The complications and management of thyroid disease in pregnancy

CASE II

Infection

A 20-year-old P1 + 0 Caucasian woman at 37 weeks' gestation contacted her general practitioner following a 48-hour illness characterized by fever, myalgia and abdominal pain. Her health before conception had been excellent, and her pregnancy had been otherwise uncomplicated. Five years previously she had delivered a daughter vaginally at term. Her daughter had been prevented from attending school for the preceding 4 days due to the 'flu'. No other family members or friends were known to be ill.

On visiting her home, the general practitioner found her to be markedly short of breath. She denied any chest pain but did report a non-productive cough which had been present for 24 hours. Her baby had been moving. Her temperature was 39.3°C, the blood pressure was 110/70 mmHg, the pulse rate was 105 bpm. and the respiratory rate was 24 per minute. The symphysis–fundal height was 38 cm and the uterus was non-tender. The fetal heart was heard at a rate of 150 bpm. The general practitioner was sufficiently concerned to contact the duty consultant obstetrician.

QI: If you had been contacted, which of the following would you have included in the differential diagnosis?
A: Pneumococcal pneumonia.
B: Pulmonary embolus.
C: Pre-eclampsia.
D: *Mycoplasma* pneumonia.
E: Sarcoidosis.
F: Tuberculosis.

Q2: What would be your advice to the general practitioner?
A: To quarantine the woman and all members of her family in their home to prevent spread of infection.
B: To put the patient to bed, administer oral antibiotics and review the following day.
C: To arrange an early antenatal clinic appointment to see the consultant.
D: To admit the patient to hospital as soon as possible – for assessment and treatment.

The patient was admitted to hospital and the findings of the general practitioner were confirmed, although her temperature on admission was 39.9°C.

Q3: What investigations may be helpful in establishing a diagnosis?

Initial investigations, including a white blood cell count and urine analysis, were unremarkable.

Some 12 hours after admission, the patient's cough had worsened, and in addition to a pyrexia of 40.5°C she had developed rigors. Chest radiography demonstrated a homogeneous right lower lobe opacity, and arterial blood gases on room air showed a pH of 7.41, a Po_2 of 9.5 kPa and a Pco_2 of 3.8 kPa. Six hours later she developed macules and vesicles over her face and trunk. Her husband then reported that her daughter and several classmates had contracted chickenpox earlier that day. The diagnosis of varicella with pneumonitis in pregnancy was thus established.

Q4: What is the natural history of varicella pneumonitis in pregnancy?

Q5: How would you manage this patient?

Her condition continued to deteriorate, and she was transferred to the intensive care unit. A repeat chest radiograph demonstrated diffuse infiltrates in all lung fields. Arterial blood gases on 40% oxygen showed a pH of 7.43, a Po_2 of 7.8 kPa and a Pco_2 of 3.7 kPa. Her respiratory rate was rapidly increasing. Parenteral acyclovir and antibiotic therapy was administered. The patient was intubated and intermittent positive-pressure ventilation was commenced. Fifty per cent oxygen with 10 cm of positive end-expiratory pressure was required. A fetal heart rate tracing was satisfactory.

Some 24 hours later, she began to labour, and after 6 hours a Neville–Barnes forceps delivery of a 2.93 kg female infant was performed. The infant was delivered in good condition, and was transferred to an isolation room on the special care baby unit.

Q6: Which of the following conditions is the female infant at an increased risk of?
A: Microphthalmia and chorioretinitis.
B: Neonatal chickenpox.
C: Microcephaly.
D: Intrauterine growth restriction.
E: Hypoplasia of limb bud development.

Q7: What would be your recommended treatment for the newborn infant?

After delivery, the patient was continued on antiviral chemotherapy for 2 weeks. Her respiratory condition gradually improved and she was extubated on the fourth postpartum day. Her daughter received varicella zoster immune globulin shortly after delivery. Both mother and daughter were discharged home in a healthy condition with no apparent sequelae.

Q8: What would have been your advice if the pregnant woman had contracted herpes zoster?

COMMENTARY

The differential diagnosis at the time of initial presentation involved determining the cause of fever and interstitial pneumonitis. The most likely cause was a respiratory infection, with the patient's daughter the probable source of infection. Given the comparatively high temperature and the apparent absence of pulmonary parenchymal consolidation, a viral infection (for example, coxsackievirus, influenza or varicella) was most likely. Alternatively, tuberculosis or the most common community-acquired bacterial pneumonia, pneumococcal pneumonia, may initially present in this fashion. Another bacterial pneumonia that might present largely as an interstitial process is that caused by *Mycoplasma pneumoniae*. The differential diagnosis should also include non-infective aetiologies such as pulmonary embolus, sarcoidosis and some collagen vascular diseases (**Q1: true = A, B, D, E, F; false = C**).

The inclusion of life-threatening conditions in the differential diagnosis (for example, the maternal mortality rate in varicella pneumonia is 2% (Paryani and Arvin, 1986)) clearly necessitates inpatient assessment and management (**Q2: true = D; false = A, B, C**).

A total and differential white blood count should be performed; a high neutrophil polymorph leucocytosis favours bacterial infection. Direct smear examination of sputum by Gram and Ziehl–Neelsen stains may give an immediate indication of possible pathogens; in pneumococcal infections Gram-staining of sputum samples shows polymorphonuclear leucocytes in addition to lancet-shaped Gram-positive diplococci. Culture of sputum samples and sensitivity testing should be carried out. Blood culture should also be performed, and may yield a positive result when sputum examination is negative. There is a variety of neutralization and complement fixation tests that may establish the serological diagnosis of viral infection, but the plethora of different viral strains makes testing for all serovarieties cumbersome, and the identification of a viral infection is often made on clinical or epidemiological grounds. Specific serological studies are probably the best method of excluding *M. pneumoniae*. A chest radiograph and skin test should exclude tuberculosis. Depending on the patient's subsequent progress, radiological studies, pleural or lymph node biopsies, and serological testing for antinuclear antibodies (or other autoimmune markers) might be indicated (**Q3**).

Almost all cases of varicella produce characteristic skin lesions, thus this diagnosis is usually established clinically. Elliptical macules, papules and fragile vesicles appear in the same dermatome. Classically, the spots appear in crops, so that lesions at all stages of development are seen simultaneously. Varicella virus can be isolated from vesicular fluid and immunological tests for varicella-specific Ig M are also reliable.

The typical clinical course of varicella pneumonitis is of a fulminant bilateral interstitial pneumonitis, which usually coincides with development of the rash. Respiratory failure is often rapid and profound.

Labour often ensues; it is unclear whether this is due to an intrauterine infection or a result of the pyrexia and severe constitutional illness (**Q4**). The patient may need intensive respiratory support and antiviral chemotherapy, and should be transferred if necessary. Intravenous acyclovir can be life saving in this situation. Although not licensed for use in pregnancy, there is an extensive register of cases where it has been used to treat pregnant women, and no long-term ill-effects have been detected thus far, in either mother or child (e.g. Hankins *et al*, 1987). The patient must be strictly isolated from staff and patients who may be susceptible to infection (**Q5**).

Skin loss and scarring, hypoplasia of skin bud development, central nervous system complications (microcephaly, cortical and cerebellar atrophy), eye complications (microphthalmia, chorioretinitis and cataracts), intrauterine growth restriction and psychomotor retardation are all potential consequences of congenital varicella syndrome, a rare complication that arises in 2–10% of cases of maternal chickenpox contracted in the first trimester of pregnancy (DeNicola and Hanshaw, 1979; Paryani and Arvin, 1986) (and thus not pertinent in this case). The baby is at risk of neonatal chickenpox. If maternal infection occurs at the end of pregnancy, the baby may be born before the mother has had time to mount an immune response and to transfer immunity, in the form of antibodies, across the placenta. Babies whose mothers develop clinical signs of infection in the last 5 days preceding or the first 2 days following delivery may acquire infection by transplacental spread associated with maternal viraemia (**Q6: true = B; false = A, C, D, E**). This illness is associated with a mortality rate of up to 30%. All at-risk babies should be given varicella zoster immune globulin (VZIG, 250 mg intramuscularly) immediately after birth, which will attenuate, but not prevent, neonatal disease. Some authors also advocate prophylactic administration of acyclovir. Separation of mother and baby is not recommended, as there is no evidence that this reduces the risk of neonatal infection. It is important to remember that all products of conception are potentially infectious, and should be handled only by those known to be immune to varicella (**Q7**).

The development of herpes zoster in a pregnant woman does not represent a particular problem to either mother or baby. The complications of herpes zoster in pregnancy are similar to those in non-pregnant women. The fetus will be protected from varicella zoster virus infection, as herpes zoster is a manifestation of reactivation, thus the mother would have passed antibodies across the placenta (**Q8**).

REFERENCES

DeNicola LK, Hanshaw JB. Congenital and neonatal varicella. *J Paediatr* 1979; **94**: 175–176.

Hankins GD, Gilstrap LC, Patterson AR. Acyclovir treatment of varicella pneumonia in pregnancy. *Crit Care Med* 1987; **15**: 336–337.

Paryani SG, Arvin AM. Intrauterine infection with varicella-zoster virus after maternal varicella. *New Engl J Med* 1986; **314**: 1542–1546.

FACTS YOU SHOULD HAVE LEARNT . . .

▶ The differential diagnosis of fever and pneumonitis
▶ The management of a pregnant woman with fever and pneumonitis
▶ The natural history of varicella in pregnancy
▶ The management of varicella in pregnancy

CASE 12

Intrauterine growth restriction

A 29-year-old P0+0 Caucasian married woman booked in her first pregnancy at 14 weeks' gestation. A blood pressure of 140/80 mmHg had been recorded at 7 weeks' gestation by her general practitioner. Her mother was known to be receiving treatment for hypertension but she had never been hypertensive and had no history of renal disease. No other problems were identified and routine antenatal care was organized with the primary care team in the community.

Q1: Is a blood pressure of 140/80 mm Hg normal for a woman of this age when 7 weeks' pregnant?

The pregnancy progressed normally until 30 weeks' gestation when the patient was admitted to hospital following a routine antenatal visit with the community midwife, when her blood pressure was 150/110 mmHg with 1+ of protein on urinalysis. She was asymptomatic and her baby was active. On abdominal examination, the symphyseal–fundal height of 27 cm was small for the gestational age.

Q2: What investigations would you perform?

An ultrasound scan showed a fetus with the abdominal circumference of 23.4 mm just above, and the head circumference and femur length just below, two standard deviations from the mean for gestation. The amniotic fluid was normal and the cardiotocograph was normal for this gestation. Doppler umbilical artery waveform analysis showed absent end-diastolic flow and the Resistance Index was 0.96. A 24-hour urine collection revealed a creatinine clearance of 115 ml per minute and a protein excretion rate of 540 mg per 24 hours. The haemoglobin level was 12.2 g dl^{-1}, the platelet count was 232×10^9 l^{-1} and the serum urate concentration was 222 μmol l^{-1}.

Q3: What are your comments about the Doppler umbilical artery waveform analysis in this case?

Q4: Does this woman have pre-eclampsia?

Q5: Which of the following treatment options would you advise at this stage?
A: Methyldopa 250 mg three times a day, discharge and review in the antenatal clinic.
B: Emergency Caesarean section.

C: Twice-daily cardiotocography with immediate delivery if any abnormality.

D: Amniocentesis to assess lung maturity.

E: Maternal intramuscular steroid treatment and monitoring of maternal and fetal well-being.

Over the following days the patient remained well and the baby was active. Her blood pressure remained at about 150/100 mmHg with 1+ of protein on urinalysis. Urine culture revealed an *Escherichia coli* infection and she was treated with the appropriate antibiotics according to sensitivities. One week later the Doppler umbilical artery waveform analysis was repeated. The Resistance Index was 0.81 and diastolic flow was noted in the umbilical arteries.

Q6: **What other forms of fetal surveillance are available to help monitor this pregnancy?**

Q7: **Which of the following statements are correct?**

A: Resistance index normally increases with advancing gestation.

B: Routine Doppler umbilical artery waveform analysis is a useful predictive test of intrauterine growth restriction.

C: The AB ratio is the most useful Doppler parameter for predicting fetal outcome.

D: A biophysical profile score of 4/10 is associated with a perinatal mortality rate of approximately 90 per 1000 births.

E: Absent diastolic flow in Doppler umbilical artery waveform analysis at 30 weeks' gestation is a definite indication to deliver the infant.

At 32 weeks' gestation the protein excretion rate was 2.01 g per day with a negative urine culture, and the patient's blood pressure was 150/90 mmHg. A repeat Doppler waveform analysis of the umbilical artery revealed no flow in diastole, and an ultrasound scan revealed little fetal growth and a liquor volume of 2.4 cm (largest pool). The platelet count and liver function test results remained normal.

Q8: **What is/are the diagnosis/es and what treatment would you advise?**

Q9: **What are the potential risks to the neonate after delivery?**

After consultation with the neonatologists the patient underwent a Caesarean section with regional anaesthesia. A baby girl was delivered who weighed 1.14 kg. There was little or no liquor noted at delivery and the umbilical vein pH was 7.32 with a base excess of 0.2 mEq l^{-1}. The baby was admitted to the neonatal unit and required 10% dextrose intravenously to maintain her blood sugar level. She commenced oral feeds on day 3 but developed right middle lobe consolidation which required intravenous antibiotic therapy for 5 days. The baby did not need respiratory support and did not develop necrotizing enterocolitis.

The mother recovered well from the operation and the hypertension resolved shortly after delivery. At the 6-week postnatal visit her daughter weighed 2.2 kg, was breastfed and was thriving.

> **Q10: What advice would you give the mother and her general practitioner regarding her future care?**

COMMENTARY

In a recent study of antenatal care, the mean blood pressure for normal women booking in the first trimester of pregnancy was 100/60 mmHg with a standard deviation of 10/8.8 mmHg (Sikorski *et al*, 1996). It is accepted that results within two standard deviations from the mean should be classified as normal; therefore the upper limit of the normal would be 130/79 mmHg (three standard deviations = 140/90 mmHg). Therefore this woman's blood pressure was abnormal. The first trimester blood pressure is an extremely useful value to help manage any subsequent rise in blood pressure in the third trimester and to distinguish physiological from pathological blood pressure readings (**Q1**).

In the presence of hypertension and proteinuria, pre-eclampsia has to be excluded by quantification of the total protein excretion over 24 hours. A urine culture must be organized to exclude urinary tract infection. Other tests that would help to assess a potential diagnosis of pre-eclampsia are a platelet count, liver function tests and estimation of serum urate levels. (Pre-eclampsia is discussed further in case 20.) Determination of the creatinine clearance rate could help exclude any pre-existing renal disease and, arguably, this should have been performed at the booking visit. With a clinical suspicion of intrauterine growth restriction, an ultrasonographic assessment of fetal size and liquor volume, and Doppler studies of the umbilical artery waveform, would be helpful (**Q2**).

The Doppler umbilical artery waveform analysis in this case appears to indicate more severe placental insufficiency than the clinical scenario would suggest and may indicate that the test should be repeated again before any decision to deliver is contemplated, as it is known that the results may be variable (**Q3**).

A diagnosis of pre-eclampsia cannot be made because a urinary tract infection has not been ruled out as possible cause of proteinuria. This is mandatory to make the diagnosis and was a serious omission. If the urine culture was negative, the diagnosis would have been secured (**Q4**).

As a consequence of this omission, none of the treatment options was appropriate. If the diagnosis of pre-eclampsia had been confirmed then maternal intramuscular steroid treatment and maternal and fetal monitoring would have been the correct option. Oral antihypertensive agents are not indicated at this level of systolic blood pressure and may compromise placental perfusion pressure. This case does not warrant immediate delivery as the mother and baby are not seriously compromised but an *in utero* transfer at this stage may well be indicated. Cardiotocographs are difficult to interpret at this gestation and the mother felt adequate fetal movements. Twice-daily cardiotocography is probably of no value. Computerized analysis of the cardiotocograph with a system like the Sonicaid System 8002 may be of value in predicting fetal acidosis and death using calculated parameters like short-term variability. Amniocentesis to obtain a lecithin/sphingomyelin ratio as an assessment of lung maturity contributes little to clinical management and the test is rarely used in the UK (**Q5: true = E; false = A, B, C, D**).

Other forms of fetal surveillance include simple observations like maternal recording of fetal activity. Biophysical profiles (a score based on ultrasonographic measurement of fetal heart rate, tone, breathing movements, body movements and liquor volume) can reflect increasing risk of perinatal mortality. (The biophysical profile is discussed in case 16.) Placental function tests (oestriol and human placental lactogen) have been discarded due to low specificities and sensitivities (**Q6**).

It has been observed that the flow in diastole with Doppler umbilical artery waveform analysis can vary; however, absent end-diastolic flow has a sensitivity of 67% and a specificity of 98% for the prediction of fetal or neonatal death. The relative risk of fetal or neonatal death with absent end-diastolic flow is increased 30-fold. The Growth Restriction Intervention Trial is currently recruiting patients to assess whether delivery will improve perinatal outcome in the absent end-diastolic flow with Doppler umbilical artery waveform analysis. With a biophysical profile score of less than six, the sensitivity for predicting fetal or neonatal death is 57% and the specificity is 91%, and the relative risk of fetal or neonatal death is increased by sixfold. A biophysical profiles score of 4/10 is associated with a high probability of fetal asphyxia, and a perinatal mortality rate of 91 per 1000 (**Q7: true = D; false = A, B, C, E**).

The diagnosis of pre-eclampsia has now been confirmed and the fetus is showing signs of compromise and may well be developing metabolic acidosis. Delivery of the fetus is indicated (**Q8**).

The main neonatal risks are associated with the problems of prematurity. These include hyaline membrane lung disease, hypothermia, hypoglycaemia, necrotizing enterocolitis, cerebral and pulmonary haemorrhage, and infection (**Q9**).

The mother and her general practitioner must be made aware of the risk of developing hypertension with advancing age. Ideally she should have her blood pressure measured yearly. The combined oral contraceptive pill should be avoided, especially combinations containing norgestrel and its C19 derivatives; for example, ethinyloestradiol 30 µg plus levonorgestrel 150 µg can alter lipid profiles adversely and predispose to arterial disease especially in the presence of hypertension. There may be a case for recommending the desogestrel and gestodene-containing oral contraceptive which have a beneficial lipid profile (Guillebraud, 1995). However, these preparations carry an increased risk of venous thrombosis, and the risks and benefits of pregnancy avoidance need to be discussed. If treatment for hypertension is necessary then angiotensin-converting enzyme inhibitors should be avoided in women of childbearing age because of the teratogenicity. Currently there are no effective methods of preventing a recurrence of pre-eclampsia or intrauterine growth restriction in any future pregnancy. Subsequent pregnancies should be monitored for fetal growth and a vaginal delivery could be contemplated (**Q10**).

REFERENCES

Guillebraud J. Advising women on which pill to take. *BMJ* 1995; **311**: 1111–1112.

Sikorski J, Wilson J, Clement S, Das S, Smeeton N. A randomised controlled trial comparing two schedules of antenatal visits: the antenatal care project. *BMJ* 1996; **312**: 546–553.

FACTS YOU SHOULD HAVE LEARNT . . .

▶ The appropriate investigations in pre-eclampsia
▶ The different methods of assessing fetal well-being
▶ The neonatal complications of premature delivery

CASE 13

Leukaemia

A 32-year-old Caucasian nulliparous woman attended the antenatal clinic at 31 weeks' gestation. She complained of lethargy but was otherwise asymptomatic. Apart from a threatened miscarriage at 6 weeks' gestation her pregnancy had been unremarkable. A detailed 19-week ultrasound scan had shown no fetal abnormality, and routine blood tests (including a full blood count at 16 weeks' gestation) had been normal. Her past medical history was unremarkable, and she was taking no medication apart from iron and folate supplementation.

A full blood count revealed a pancytopenia with marked neutropenia (haemoglobin 9.5 g dl^{-1}, platelet count 121 × 10^9 l^{-1}, white cell count 1.1 × 10^9 l^{-1}, neutrophils 0.2 × 10^9 l^{-1}).

Q1: **Which of the following statements regarding haematological indices in pregnancy are correct?**
A: Both the platelet count and the mean platelet volume fall in normal pregnancies.
B: A white cell count of 1.1 × 10^9 l^{-1} in the third trimester is within two standard deviations of the mean.
C: The haematocrit falls in normal pregnancy.
D: In pregnant women given prophylactic iron and folate supplementation, the mean cell haemoglobin concentration falls in pregnancy.

The blood film showed basophilic stippling and polychromasia. A coagulation screen was normal. Fibrinogen degradation products were raised at 2.0 g l^{-1} (normal value < 0.5 g l^{-1}), but the plasma fibrinogen level was normal. A preliminary diagnosis of leukaemia was made, and the patient was referred to a consultant haematologist.

Q2: **When you counsel the patient, which of the following are accurate statements?**
A: The incidence of leukaemia is increased in pregnancy.
B: Most leukaemias in pregnancy are acute leukaemias.
C: The diagnosis of leukaemia should be confirmed by bone marrow biopsy and aspirate.
D: Treatment should be instigated as quickly as possible.
E: Transmission of maternal malignant cells to the fetus is extremely rare.

After referral to the haematology department, a bone marrow aspirate and trephine were taken from the iliac crest. This showed the diagnosis to be acute promyelocytic leukaemia (French–American–British classification M-3) with 60% of nucleated cells being promyelocytes or blasts. This was confirmed after urgent cytogenetics revealed the 15/17 translocation classically seen in acute promyelocytic leukaemia (APL): 46XX t{15 : 17 } {q22 : q11}.

Q3: **When considering the most appropriate treatment, which of the following are accurate statements?**

A: The standard treatment for acute leukaemia is combination cytotoxic chemotherapy.

B: Delivery of the baby at this gestation would involve minimal risk to mother or baby.

C: If undelivered, risks of cytotoxic therapy to the baby include intrauterine growth restriction and preterm labour.

D: Risks of cytotoxic therapy to the mother include reduced fertility.

Q4: **What treatment would you recommend? Is there a reasonable alternative to delivery and commencement of cytotoxic therapy?**

It was decided to treat the patient with differential induction therapy, using all-trans retinoic acid (ATRA) at an oral dose of 45 $mg\,m^{-2}$. An ultrasound scan was performed before initiating ATRA treatment to obtain baseline measurements for monitoring fetal growth. After commencing ATRA there was a rapid improvement in haematological indices, with the white cell count rising to normal levels within 2 weeks. After a transfusion of 2 units of packed red cells, a haemoglobin concentration of 10.5 $g\,dl^{-1}$ was attained. Coagulation screens remained normal, as did renal and liver function test results, although the lactate dehydrogenase level did show a moderate rise with treatment. Serial ultrasound scans confirmed good growth of a normal-sized fetus.

At 35 weeks' gestation, analysis of a repeat bone marrow biopsy confirmed complete morphological remission and normal cytogenetics.

Q5: **When would you plan to deliver the baby?**

Q6: **When considering labour and delivery, which of the following are accurate statements?**

A: Elective Caesarean section is the optimal mode of delivery.

B: An epidural is contraindicated.

C: Antibiotic prophylaxis should be given.

After discussion, delivery was planned for 36 weeks. The decision to aim for a vaginal delivery was made; the patient was entirely asymptomatic, and the presenting part was cephalic and close to engagement. She was admitted for prostaglandin induction of labour, and, after cervical ripening, the membranes were ruptured artificially and a Syntocinon infusion was commenced. An epidural was sited 3 hours after the membranes were ruptured, and after a further 2 hours the cervix was found to be fully dilated. At this time the cardiotocograph displayed some late decelerations. Delivery was thus expedited using the ventouse. A healthy female infant with a birthweight of 2480 g (10th centile at

36 weeks' gestation) was delivered with good Apgar scores. The baby had no congenital abnormalities and the newborn examination was normal. Blood loss at delivery was minimal.

Mother and baby made good progress and were discharged home 3 days following delivery, with the mother continuing ATRA therapy which was interrupted for only 24 hours around the time of delivery. A full blood count taken 6 days after delivery was satisfactory (haemoglobin 11.2 $g\,dl^{-1}$, platelet count $443 \times 10^9\,l^{-1}$, white cell count $11.7 \times 10^9\,l^{-1}$, neutrophils $8.8 \times 10^9\,l^{-1}$). At a 3-week check, the infant was found to be making normal progress in terms of both growth and development, with no ill effects consequent upon the ATRA therapy. The mother was readmitted under the care of haematologists for intensive combination chemotherapy 2 weeks after the delivery.

Q7: What is the overall chance of recovery for this patient?

COMMENTARY

Pregnancy is associated with diminutions in the red blood cell count, haemoglobin concentration, haematocrit, platelet count and a rise in the mean platelet volume. The values of the mean red cell volume, mean cell haemoglobin and mean cell haemoglobin concentration in the third trimester approximate to those of non-pregnant women. When women receive prophylactic iron and folate supplementation, the values of the red blood cell count, haemoglobin concentration and haematocrit fall in the first trimester. However, when supplementation is given, there are no further pregnancy-related reductions in these indices. In the third trimester of pregnancy, the mean total white cell count is approximately $10.2 \times 10^9\,l^{-1}$, with a standard deviation of $3.4 \times 10^9\,l^{-1}$ (non-pregnant values $5.6 \pm 1.0 \times 10^9\,l^{-1}$). A value of $1.1 \times 10^9\,l^{-1}$ is thus well below two standard deviations from the mean (**Q1: true = C; false = A, B, D**).

The annual incidence of leukaemia in pregnancy is about one case per 75 000 pregnancies, with most cases being diagnosed in the second or third trimesters. Approximately 50% of cases are of acute leukaemia, with acute myeloid leukaemia being commoner than acute lymphoblastic (in a ratio of about 2:1). Transmission of maternal malignant cells to the fetus is extremely rare, and there is no evidence that the incidence of leukaemia is increased in or by pregnancy. However, a delay in diagnosis can occur because of confusion of symptoms with those of normal pregnancy (breathlessness, lethargy, anaemia). Any delay in instigating treatment can threaten maternal and fetal survival, as untreated patients have a median survival of only 2 months (**Q2: true = C, D, E; false = A, B**).

Acute promyelocytic leukaemia (APL) is a unique and important subset of acute myeloid leukaemia, and is characterized by:

► Neoplastic proliferation of promyelocytes (the precursors of neutrophils),

> a specific chromosomal translocation (t{15 : 17}), and
> a high incidence of disseminated intravascular coagulation (DIC).

As DIC is often exacerbated by both pregnancy and by conventional cytotoxic therapy, APL is a potentially life-threatening situation which requires careful management.

The standard treatment for APL is aggressive chemotherapy which is harmful to the fetus. Risks to the fetus include increased rates of miscarriage, teratogenicity, intrauterine growth restriction and preterm labour, in addition to long-term risks such as poor infant growth, diminished intellectual capacity, reduced immunological status, increased risk of childhood cancers and reduced fertility. Risks to the mother result from bone marrow suppression, with altered haemostasis and a danger of overwhelming infection. Although fertility may be reduced, the younger the woman at the time of diagnosis and treatment, the greater the chance that fertility will be retained. On the other hand, delivery of the baby at this gestation would have been harmful to both the mother in her pancytopenic state (especially secondary to haemorrhage and infection) and the fetus, which would be at considerable risk of developing complications of prematurity such as hyaline membrane disease (**Q3: true = A, C, D; false = B**).

ATRA (all-trans retinoic acid) is a vitamin A derivative which has been successfully used to induce remission in APL (use since 1988 has established that ATRA successfully induces a response in over 95% of cases). When administered in the first trimester of pregnancy, retinoids are strongly associated with miscarriage and teratogenicity (thus women taking retinoic acid for acne need careful contraceptive counselling). Miscarriage rates of 20–40%, and rates of major malformations of 25–35%, have been reported. There have been no reports of retinoid-related problems in the second or third trimesters of pregnancy. ATRA is administered orally and induces maturation of immature promyelocytes into mature neutrophils. The response to ATRA is rapid, with complete remission being attained within 6 weeks of therapy, and is associated with a rapid improvement in haemostatic disorders with no bone marrow suppression. ATRA was first used successfully to treat APL in a pregnant woman in 1993. It was used in a woman who had developed APL at 26 weeks' gestation, and complete remission was induced before an elective Caesarean section at 30 weeks' gestation (Harrison et al, 1994) (**Q4**).

At 36 weeks' gestation it was considered that the risks of further delaying intensive chemotherapy (including the psychological morbidity of the patient and her husband who were awaiting the potentially curative treatment) outweighed the risks to the fetus of prematurity (**Q5**).

With the fetal head engaged and at 36 weeks' gestation, it was reasonable to attempt a vaginal delivery in order to avoid the morbidity of a Caesarean section. As the patient was in remission there was no contraindication to epidural anaesthesia (haematological investigations were normal) and no necessity for antibiotic prophylaxis (**Q6: all false**).

The combined cytotoxic treatment carries an overall chance of recovery of approximately 70% (**Q7**).

REFERENCE

Harrison P, Chipping P, Fothergill GA. Successful use of ATRA in APL presenting during the second trimester of pregnancy. *Br J Haematol* 1994; **86**: 681–682.

FACTS YOU SHOULD HAVE LEARNT . . .

▶ The pregnancy-related changes in haematological indices
▶ The diagnosis, management and prognosis of a woman with acute leukaemia in pregnancy

CASE 14

A low platelet count

A 22-year-old para $0+1$ woman attended the hospital antenatal booking clinic at 18 weeks' gestation. Her past medical history was unremarkable, and a detailed ultrasound scan did not reveal any abnormality (fetal measurements were consistent with the date of her last menstrual period). A full blood count was subsequently reported as having demonstrated a platelet count of $76 \times 10^9 \ 1^{-1}$; all other parameters were normal. She was asked to reattend the antenatal clinic.

Q1: **What is your definition of thrombocytopenia, and what is the incidence in pregnancy?**

Q2: **Which of the following should be included in the differential diagnosis?**
A: Pre-eclampsia.
B: Idiopathic/autoimmune thrombocytopenic purpura (AITP).
C: Systemic lupus erythematosus (SLE).
D: Folic acid deficiency.
E: Thrombotic thrombocytopenic purpura (TTP).
F: Prolonged retention of a dead fetus.

Q3: **When the patient reattends the clinic, what features of the history and examination would you recheck?**

Examination of a stained blood film revealed the presence of megathrombocytes (younger, larger platelets), and the mean platelet volume was above the normal range. Immunological tests for antinuclear antibody, anticardiolipin antibody and lupus anticoagulant were negative.

Q4: **Which of the following tests would you wish to perform?**
A: A bone marrow aspiration biopsy.
B: A coagulation profile.
C: Antiplatelet antibody estimation.
D: Measurement of platelet-associated immunoglobulin IgG.

A diagnosis of AITP was made, and the possibility of the baby suffering problems due to a low platelet count was discussed with the patient (although the fact that this risk was low in the absence of a history of AITP before the pregnancy was stressed). She was reviewed in the hospital antenatal clinic every 4 weeks, and reviewed jointly by an obstetrician and a haematologist. She remained asymptomatic and the pregnancy was otherwise uncomplicated. At 24 weeks' gestation the platelet count was

65×10^9 l^{-1}, and at 28 weeks' gestation the count was 62×10^9 l^{-1}. However, at 32 weeks' gestation a count of 43×10^9 l^{-1} was recorded, and a decision to prescribe a 3-week course of prednisolone 10 mg per day was made.

Q5: What are the problems of steroid therapy in pregnancy?

Despite prednisolone therapy, her platelet count did not rise, and was 40×10^9 l^{-1} at 35 weeks' gestation. A decision was made to administer a 50 g intravenous IgG infusion at 36 weeks' gestation.

Q6: What are the advantages and disadvantages of an IgG infusion?

Q7: What alternative treatments might have resulted in an increased platelet count?

Two days after the IgG infusion, the platelet count was rechecked and was found to be 92×10^9 l^{-1}.

Q8: In deciding the mode of delivery for a patient with AITP, which of the following statements are correct?
   A: The risk of severe fetal thrombocytopenia at term (platelet count $< 50 \times 10^9$ l^{-1}) is not more than 5%.
   B: Fetal scalp sampling in labour is a useful adjunct to a decision regarding mode of delivery.
   C: In cases of AITP, Caesarean section is the optimal mode of delivery.
   D: If the fetus is known to have severe fetal thrombocytopenia (platelet count $< 50 \times 10^9$ l^{-1}), a Caesarean section has been proved to be the optimal mode of delivery.

In this case, a breech presentation was found on examination in the antenatal clinic at 36 weeks' gestation, and on an ultrasound scan the fetus was found to have a flexed breech presentation and an estimated weight of 3.2 kg. After discussion of the different options, the patient was adamant that she wished to deliver by elective Caesarean section. On admission at 38 weeks' gestation, before the Caesarean section, the platelet count was 96×10^9 l^{-1}, and the coagulation profile was normal. Platelets were available but were not given prophylactically.

Q9: Is an epidural a safe form of anaesthetic?

A 3.41 kg male infant was delivered in good condition at Caesarean section. The platelet count in the umbilical vein was 187×10^9 l^{-1}.

Q10: In pregnancies complicated by AITP, when is the baby at greatest risk?

A follow-up neonatal platelet count 2 days later was 185×10^9 l^{-1}. Neither mother nor baby suffered complications, and both were discharged on the fifth postoperative day.

COMMENTARY

The normal platelet count during pregnancy is $150-350 \times 10^9 \text{ l}^{-1}$, although a threshold of counts below $100 \times 10^9 \text{ l}^{-1}$ is usually considered to reflect significant thrombocytopenia. With the increased availability of automated platelet counting, the unexpected discovery of thrombocytopenia in an otherwise healthy pregnant woman has become relatively common, and 5–10% of pregnant women have a platelet count below $150 \times 10^9 \text{ l}^{-1}$ at some time during their pregnancy (**Q1**).

There are a number of clinically significant thrombocytopenic disorders that may adversely effect the mother and fetus. These include conditions that are specific to pregnancy and those coincidental to pregnancy. Management and prognosis vary with the aetiology, thus it is important to establish a diagnosis. Causes of thrombocytopenia in pregnancy include pre-eclampsia, disseminated intravascular coagulation (DIC) (secondary to conditions such as placental abruption, amniotic fluid embolism and prolonged retention of a dead fetus), AITP, SLE or other connective tissue disorders, TTP, and primary bone marrow failure of any aetiology. By definition, pre-eclampsia is a diagnosis of the second half of pregnancy and is therefore not relevant to this case. Thrombocytopenia is seen only as a consequence of a severe megaloblastic picture due to folic acid deficiency in association with low white cell counts and macrocytosis. The otherwise normal full blood count also makes a diagnosis of TTP unlikely (the pentad of pyrexia, haemolytic anaemia, neurological disorder, renal dysfunction and thrombocytopenia is pathognomonic for TTP). An ultrasound scan had demonstrated fetal viability at the time of the full blood count (**Q2: true = B, C; false = A, D, E, F**).

The patient's medical and family history should be reviewed in detail for diagnoses associated with low platelet counts such as SLE or AITP. Has she undergone splenectomy? Has she had a recent infection, haematuria, menorrhagia, epistaxis, transfusion or noted bruising. Is she taking any medication that might contribute to thrombocytopenia? The physical examination should be comprehensive and include a search for ecchymoses, petechiae and purpura (**Q3**).

In most cases, a history, examination and full blood count will establish a diagnosis of AITP. A bone marrow aspiration biopsy is rarely necessary for thrombocytopenia in pregnancy. The procedure is uncomfortable, risky and, whilst it may demonstrate an abundance of megakaryocytes, this can be deduced from the peripheral film. Its major use should be the detection of infiltrative marrow disease, and thus it should be considered only if the platelet count is much lower. Although bleeding problems are uncommon unless the platelet count is below $50 \times 10^9 \text{ l}^{-1}$, a coagulation profile is probably appropriate. Although AITP is caused by circulating antiplatelet autoantibodies (APAs), estimation of APA has not been consistently predictive of either haemorrhage or neonatal platelet count. Measurement of platelet-associated IgG (PAIgG) is a direct test to quantify the antibody bound to tested platelets. However, direct PAIgG is not a specific test for

AITP and does not correlate with neonatal platelet counts or the risk of fetal or neonatal haemorrhage (**Q4: true = probably B; false = probably A, C, D**).

An association between steroid administration and cleft lips or palates has been suggested. Side-effects for the mother include weight gain, subcutaneous fat redistribution and hypertension. The prevalence of pre-eclampsia, gestational diabetes, puerperal psychosis and osteoporosis are all increased by steroid therapy. Such treatment should thus be reserved for patients with symptoms or with platelet counts below $50 \times 10^9 \, l^{-1}$. Suppression of the fetal adrenal glands is a theoretical hazard, but over 90% of prednisolone is metabolized in the placenta and thus never reaches the fetus (**Q5**).

Administration of monomeric polyvalent human IgG in doses greater than those produced endogenously prolongs the clearance time of immune complexes by the reticuloendothelial system, and this results in an increase in the number of circulating platelets. A dose of $0.4 \, g \, kg^{-1}$ for 5 days was originally recommended, but alternative regimens that are easier to manage and use less total immunoglobulin have been suggested (Burrows and Kelton, 1992). A typical dose is $1 \, g \, kg^{-1}$ over 8 hours; the dose can be repeated 2 days later if the platelet count does not rise appropriately. The advantages of IgG infusions are that there are few side-effects and the response is both more reliable and more rapid than that with steroid treatment. The response usually occurs within 48 hours and is maintained for up to 3 weeks. IgG infusions do not provide a long-term cure for AITP, and the other disadvantage relates to the cost of this therapy. Initial suggestions that IgG can cross the placenta and provoke similar responses in the fetus have not been proven; exogenous IgG may not even cross the placenta (**Q6**).

Other methods of increasing the platelet count include a platelet transfusion, although this would usually be considered only in a symptomatic patient. Splenectomy will produce a cure or long-term remission in about 70% of patients with AITP. Although removal of the spleen remains an option if all other attempts to increase the platelet count fail, splenectomy is rarely indicated in a pregnant woman and should be avoided given the success of medical management. Other drugs that have been used successfully in the treatment of AITP, such as danazol, vincristine and cyclophosphamide, are contraindicated in pregnancy (**Q7**).

There is little risk to the mother whatever mode of delivery is chosen. The major risk is to the fetus with thrombocytopenia, who may suffer intracranial haemorrhage as a result of birth trauma. Fetal scalp sampling in labour was suggested as a direct and timely test of fetal platelet count. However, the deliberate laceration of the scalp of a baby suspected to have a coagulopathy is cause for concern. Moreover, correlation with neonatal platelet count and with the likelihood of haemorrhage is poor, thus this procedure is no longer advocated. Based on an estimated perinatal mortality rate approaching 20%, it was proposed that Caesarean section should be performed in all pregnancies complicated by AITP (Murray and

Harris, 1987). However, the cases analysed were severely symptomatic, and this rate is a gross overestimate. A recent comprehensive review found that perinatal and neonatal mortality rates were only marginally increased, and that all the deaths occurred in babies delivered by Caesarean section (Burrows and Kelton, 1992). Because the risk of severe fetal thrombocytopenia at term (platelet count $< 50 \times 10^9 \, l^{-1}$) is not more than 5%, and because the reduction in neonatal morbidity and mortality by prophylactic Caesarean section has not been demonstrated, delivery by Caesarean section should be reserved for cases with obstetric indication. The utility of intrauterine umbilical blood sampling is not yet clear, but has been advocated in women who have needed treatment for AITP. Proponents deliver any fetus with significant thrombocytopenia by elective Caesarean section, but it should be stressed that this management is arbitrary and is not based on controlled data (**Q8: true = A; false = B, C, D**).

Most anaesthetists require that the platelet count is over $80 \times 10^9 \, l^{-1}$ before they will administer an epidural anaesthetic, but there is no good evidence that counts above $50 \times 10^9 \, l^{-1}$ are not sufficient to achieve haemostasis in AITP (**Q9**).

The neonatal platelet count falls in the first few days of life, and the maximum risk period is 2–3 days after delivery. The platelet count should be repeated daily for a week in any baby with thrombocytopenia at delivery. Postpartum concerns in the mother relate to the incision, which should be inspected carefully during the postpartum period (**Q10**).

REFERENCES

Burrows RF, Kelton JG. Thrombocytopenia during pregnancy. In: Greer IA, Fornes CD (eds) *Haemostasis and Thrombosis in Obstetrics and Gynaecology*, pp. 407–429. London: Chapman & Hall, 1992.

Murray JM, Harris RE. The management of the pregnant patient with idiopathic thrombocytopenic purpura. *Am J Obstet Gynecol* 1987; **126**; 449–451.

FACTS YOU SHOULD HAVE LEARNT . . .

‣ The differential diagnosis of thrombocytopenia in pregnancy
‣ The characteristic features of autoimmune (or idiopathic) thrombocytopenic purpura
‣ The management of autoimmune thrombocytopenic purpura

CASE 15

Placenta praevia

A 25-year-old P1 + 0 woman attended the antenatal booking clinic at 18 weeks' gestation. She had previously undergone an elective lower segment Caesarean section for an anterior grade III placenta praevia. Her past medical history was otherwise unremarkable. A detailed ultrasound scan did not reveal any fetal abnormality, but indicated that the placenta covered the internal os. The patient's blood group was O Rh positive; no red cell antibodies were detected.

> **Q1:** When determining whether the planned mode of delivery should be a vaginal delivery or a repeat elective Caesarean section, which of the following are correct?
> A: The risk of uterine rupture is significantly higher in women undergoing a trial of labour with a uterine scar.
> B: Maternal morbidity is lower in women undergoing a trial of labour.
> C: Women with a history suggestive of cephalopelvic disproportion have the lowest success rate for vaginal birth after Caesarean section
> D: Multiple pregnancies should be delivered by elective Caesarean section, if a previous Caesarean section has been performed.
> E: Delivery should be by elective Caesarean section after more than one Caesarean section has been performed.

A decision to aim for a trial of labour (provided there was no placenta praevia at the time of delivery) was made.

> **Q2:** Which of the following statements relating to a trial of labour after Caesarean section are correct?
> A: Prostaglandin induction of labour is of proven danger.
> B: Augmentation of labour with oxytocin should be avoided.
> C: Regional analgesia is contraindicated.
> D: Post-partum scar palpation should be practised.

The pregnancy remained uncomplicated. When the patient reattended the hospital antenatal clinic at 34 weeks' gestation, an ultrasound examination revealed an anterior placenta praevia, with the placenta covering the internal os asymmetrically. The patient was admitted to the antenatal ward and remained an inpatient. At no time was there any vaginal bleeding.

> **Q3:** Which of the following should be regarded as risk factors for placenta praevia?
> A: Pre-eclampsia.
> B: Smoking.

C: Previous Caesarean section.
D: Nulliparity.
E: Previous placenta praevia.

Q4: **In this case, what is the grade of placenta praevia?**

Q5: **In the expectant management of placenta praevia, which of the following statements are correct?**
A: Patients should be in hospital from diagnosis to delivery.
B: Tocolytics should not be administered if preterm labour occurs.
C: Cross-matched blood should be ready at all times.
D: Perinatal mortality is directly related to the amount of blood lost antepartum.
E: Approximately 20% of women deliver before 32 weeks' gestation.

At 37 weeks' gestation, a further ultrasound scan was performed and placental localization was unchanged. Echo-planar imaging (EPI) was performed, and the EPI scan confirmed the ultrasonographic findings of anterior placenta praevia. The previous Caesarean section scar was also visualized. While the placenta was seen to overlie the scar tissue, a plane between the uterus and the placenta at this site was apparent. A morbidly adherent placenta (discussed further in case 26) was thus deemed to be unlikely.

Q6: **What other imaging methods have been used to localize the placenta?**

A Caesarean section was performed by a senior obstetrician at 38 weeks' gestation. A right-sided placenta praevia, extending over the previous scar and reaching the internal os, was noted. The placenta separated from the uterus with ease, and total blood loss was less than 500 ml. A male infant weighing 3.10 kg was delivered in good condition. The patient made an uneventful recovery and did not require a transfusion.

Q7: **Which of the following statements concerning Caesarean section for placenta praevia are correct?**
A: Placenta praevia is an absolute contraindication to regional anaesthesia.
B: The optimal uterine incision is a transverse lower segment incision.
C: An intramyometrial injection of prostaglandin $F_{2\alpha}$ should be given as prophylaxis against postpartum haemorrhage.
D: Intrapartum and postpartum haemorrhage are greater than average, because of retained products of conception.

COMMENTARY

Over the past 20 years, the medical pendulum has swung back in favour of trial of labour after Caesarean section. It is now accepted as standard obstetric practice that one previous lower segment Caesarean section is an indication for a trial of vaginal delivery in a subsequent pregnancy, provided there are no adverse risk factors. There have not been any randomized controlled trials comparing the results of elective repeat Caesarean section and trial of labour for women who have had a previous Caesarean section. However, meta-analysis of seven prospective cohort studies indicated an overall vaginal delivery rate of almost 80% of women permitted a trial of labour (Enkin, 1989). There is no significant difference in the rate of uterine dehiscence or rupture of women undergoing repeat Caesarean section and those having a trial of labour (irrespective of eventual mode of delivery) (Enkin, 1989). All measured parameters of maternal morbidity are lower in trial-of-labour groups. Women with a history of cephalopelvic disproportion have the lowest success rate for vaginal birth after Caesarean section, but still have a 50% chance of successful vaginal delivery. Attention is now turning to the appropriate delivery mode after more than one Caesarean section, or with a twin gestation. Several studies have supported the feasibility and safety of vaginal delivery in these circumstances. Of note is the absence of maternal or fetal morbidity or mortality in such labours (**Q1: true = B, C; false = A, probably D, E**).

Concern has been expressed regarding the safety of prostaglandin in cases of previous Caesarean section, because of the risk of uterine rupture. However, what little evidence that exists suggests that the use of prostaglandin gel to attain cervical ripening is effective and does not lead to uterine dehiscence. Current obstetric opinion is that a previous Caesarean section is not a contraindication to the use of oxytocin in labour. However, most practitioners would discontinue a trial of labour if a prompt response to oxytocin stimulation did not occur, and would be reticent to start oxytocin if the partogram suggested a secondary arrest pattern. Any decision regarding induction or augmentation of labour with Syntocinon should be made by a senior obstetrician. Epidural analgesia is not associated with an increased risk of or from uterine rupture. Uterine dehiscence is often asymptomatic, and even overt rupture may not be associated with classical signs of pain and tenderness, irrespective of whether regional analgesia is being used. No study has demonstrated that manual exploration of a previous Caesarean section scar is of benefit. The procedure may introduce infection or convert a small dehiscence into an overt rupture (**Q2: false =A, B, C, D**).

Although the cause of placenta praevia is unclear, various risk factors have been identified. These include age, parity, smoking, previous Caesarean sections and a previous history of placenta praevia. The recurrence risk is approximately 5% after one placenta praevia (**Q3: true = B, C, E; false = A, D**).

Four grades of placenta praevia have been defined. In grade I, the placenta is in the lower uterine segment but the lower edge does not reach the internal os. In grade II, the lower edge of the placenta reaches but does not cover the os. In grade III, the placenta covers the os asymmetrically (as in this case), and in grade IV the placenta covers the os symmetrically (**Q4**).

The expectant management of placenta praevia, as originally advocated by Macafee (1945), aims to achieve maximum fetal maturity, whilst minimizing the risks to both mother and fetus. Macafee argued that patients should remain in hospital from diagnosis to delivery. Although certain authors have subsequently suggested that selected women can return home, their selection criteria are ill defined, and the majority of obstetricians would concur that optimal expectant management incorporates inpatient hospitalization. During expectant management, 40% of women labour before 37 weeks, and 20% before 32 weeks. Inhibiting uterine activity in cases of preterm labour seems logical, but antepartum haemorrhage is a relative contraindication to tocolytic therapy as placental abruption cannot be excluded. Placental abruption coexists with placenta praevia in 10% of cases, and sympathomimetics produce maternal tachycardias and palpitations that could be confused with hypovolaemia. There is no consensus regarding tocolytic therapy, but in the opinion of the authors the advantages of steroid therapy are such that a 24-hour course of sympathomimetic therapy to enable steroid administration should be considered when patients with placenta praevia labour before 32 weeks' gestation. Perinatal mortality is directly related to the total amount of blood lost antepartum. This effect is nullified by adequate recourse to blood transfusion, and cross-matched blood must be available at all times (**Q5: true = A, C, D, E; false = probably B**).

Although ultrasonography is the mainstay of placental localization, other methods such as soft tissue placentography (using X-rays), radioisotope radiography, pelvic angiography and thermography have been used. Although the high cost of magnetic resonance imaging limits availability, it may well be a technique of the future. EPI is a form of nuclear magnetic resonance imaging with short image acquisition times. Each image is displayed in transection as it is acquired in real time. EPI has been used accurately to estimate fetal size and organ volumes (Baker *et al*, 1995). In this case EPI was used to evaluate a uterine scar and its relationship to the placenta in order to diagnose or exclude a morbidly adherent placenta. An accurate prediction of cases likely to be complicated by a morbidly adherent placenta is of benefit to patient, surgeon and anaesthetist. The patient can be counselled as to the likelihood of a Caesarean hysterectomy (discussed in case 26). Similarly, the surgeon and anaesthetist can prepare for the most appropriate operative procedure (**Q6**).

By lowering blood pressure, regional anaesthesia may critically reduce uterine and placental perfusion. However, when the patient is stable with no active bleeding, regional anaesthesia should not be regarded as contraindicated provided a senior anaesthetist is present. Even when regional anaesthesia is used, it is often appropriate to suggest that partners are not in the operating theatre, owing to the possibility of severe haemorrhage. The uterine incision should usually be a lower transverse incision. When the lower segment is barely formed or is very vascular, classical or De Lee's (lower midline) incisions have been advocated. However, complications of classical and De Lee's incisions are sufficiently high to make their use rarely warranted. Because the lower segment is less muscular than the remainder of the uterus, contraction and retraction (which occlude the sinuses of the placental bed) are inadequate, and bleeding is increased. Intramyometrial injection of prostaglandin $F_{2\alpha}$ has been used successfully in cases of excessive intrapartum and post-partum haemorrhage, but is not used as prophylactic therapy (**Q7: true = B; false = A, C, D**).

REFERENCES

Baker PN, Johnson IR, Gowland PAM et al. Measurement of fetal brain, liver and placental volumes with echoplanar magnetic resonance imaging. *Br J Obstet Gynaecol* 1995; **102**: 35–39.

Enkin M. Labour and delivery following previous Caesarean section. In: Chalmers I, Enkin M, Kierse MJNC (eds) *Effective Care in Pregnancy and Childbirth*, pp. 1196–1215. Oxford: Oxford University Press, 1989.

Macafee CHG. Placenta praevia: a study of 174 cases. *J Obstet Gynaecol Br Emp* 1945; **52**: 313–324.

FACTS YOU SHOULD HAVE LEARNT . . .

▶ **The rationale for a trial of labour after a Caesarean section**
▶ **The management of a trial of labour after a Caesarean section**
▶ **The management of placenta praevia**

CASE 16

Pruritus

A 32-year-old para 1 + 0 Caucasian woman attended the hospital antenatal booking clinic at 18 weeks' gestation. Her obstetric history was significant for a term stillbirth of unknown aetiology in her first pregnancy. In the previous pregnancy, she had been referred by her community midwife after no fetal heart was audible, and she had not noted any fetal movements for 3 days. After induction of labour, a macerated male infant weighing 2.41 kg had been delivered. The subsequent postmortem examination had found a small morphologically normal infant. Her past medical history was otherwise unremarkable, and a detailed ultrasound scan did not reveal any abnormality (fetal measurements were consistent with the date of her last menstrual period). The provisional plan was to perform serial ultrasonographic estimations of fetal growth and electively to induce delivery at 38 weeks' gestation.

When the patient was reviewed at 26 weeks' gestation, she was asymptomatic and good fetal growth was noted on both clinical examination and ultrasound scan. However, on review 4 weeks later, she gave a 2-week history of marked and distressing pruritus, which was particularly pronounced in her palms and soles. No abnormality was found on physical examination; no skin rash was present, and there was no evidence of jaundice, ascites or hepatosplenomegaly.

Q1:   In the absence of a skin rash, which of the following should be included in the differential diagnosis of pruritus?

A: Acute fatty liver of pregnancy.

B: Lymphoma.

C: Hyperplacentosis.

D: Intrahepatic cholestasis of pregnancy.

Laboratory tests revealed a haematocrit of 33.3%, a platelet count of $240 \times 10^9 \, l^{-1}$, a fibrinogen level of 320 mg dl^{-1} and normal liver enzymes. The prothrombin time and serum bilirubin level were in the upper range of normal. Serum bile acids were measured at 358 μmol l^{-1} (normally below 6 μmol l^{-1}) and urine analysis was positive for urobilinogen.

Q2:   What other investigations would you have instigated?

A diagnosis of intrahepatic cholestasis of pregnancy (ICP) was made, and further questioning revealed that the patient suffered from generalized pruritus in her previous pregnancy.

Q3:   What is intrahepatic cholestasis of pregnancy?

Q4: What is the incidence of the condition?

Q5: Which of the following conditions have an increased incidence in ICP?
A: Placental abruption.
B: Premature labour.
C: Cholelithiasis.
D: Intrapartum fetal distress.
E: Third trimester stillbirth.

Antihistamines and cholestyramine (4 g orally thrice daily) were prescribed, but the pruritus was only minimally diminished.

Q6: What other treatment options would you suggest?

When the patient reattended the hospital antenatal clinic at 34 weeks' gestation, the symphysis–fundal height was measured at 31 cm. She reported good fetal activity. Ultrasound scan measurements of fetal growth indicated that, although fetal head growth was normal (both the biparietal diameter and head circumference approximated to the 50th centile), abdominal growth was diminished, with the abdominal circumference (AC) on the 5th centile.

Q7: When considering ultrasonographic measurement of fetal growth, which of the following statements are correct?
A: The AC is the single best and most useful reflection of fetal growth.
B: The most accurate AC is the largest one obtained between fetal respirations at the level of the hepatic vein.
C: An AC below the 5th centile for gestational age indicates that the fetus is growth restricted.
D: Advantages of biparietal diameter measurements over head circumference measurements include a greater resistance to external factors (oligohydramnios or breech presentation).

A biophysical profile was performed, and a score of 10/10 was attained. However, 1 week later, when the patient presented with a history of diminished fetal movements, the biophysical profile score was 4/10.

Q8: Which of the following statements regarding biophysical profile scoring are correct?
A: A pocket of amniotic fluid greater than 3 cm is classified as normal and results in a score of 2.
B: Parameters include ultrasonographic estimation of fetal growth.
C: Fewer than three body limb movements in 30 minutes is classified as abnormal.
D: Absent end-diastolic flow is classified as abnormal and results in a score of 0.
E: The amniotic fluid volume is the most important parameter.

F: The negative predictive value (normal score, still healthy at 7 days) is greater than 99%.

G: Fetal breathing movements are the parameter most likely to be absent in an otherwise normal test.

The patient was admitted to the labour ward for induction of labour. On vaginal examination the cervix was found to be wholly unfavourable, and a 1 mg prostaglandin E_2 vaginal gel was inserted. Shortly after this insertion two fetal heart rate decelerations were noted (in the absence of detectable uterine activity), and a decision to perform a Caesarean section was made. Under spinal anaesthesia, a 2350 g male infant was delivered with an Apgar score of 5 at 1 minute and of 8 at 5 minutes. Umbilical cord artery and vein pH values were 7.22 and 7.26 respectively. The baby had no neonatal problems and they were both discharged home on the sixth postoperative day. The patient continued to complain of pruritus for about 10 days following delivery. When she was reviewed at her 6-week postnatal visit, she was asymptomatic and all laboratory tests were normal.

Q9: How would you counsel this patient regarding a possible recurrence?

COMMENTARY

There are many causes of pruritus which are associated with skin lesions; these include generalized skin conditions such as eczema and psoriasis, medication, and infections such as scabies. In the absence of dermatological abnormalities, pruritus associated with pregnancy is usually due to intrahepatic cholestasis of pregnancy (ICP), although other systemic diseases associated with pruritus include lymphoma, liver disease and thyroid dysfunction, and sometimes no cause is found. It has been suggested that an overactive placenta, as measured by raised levels of human chorionic gonadotrophin, can be a cause of pruritus, provided other conditions have been excluded. Patients with acute fatty liver of pregnancy characteristically present with vomiting, malaise and abdominal pain, followed by jaundice with drowsiness or confusion (**Q1: true = B, D, perhaps C; false = A**).

The maternal history and the markedly raised levels of bile acids, strongly suggested a diagnosis of ICP. In cases of ICP, levels of bilirubin and alkaline phosphatase are often raised, although the latter is typically increased in pregnancy. Standard liver function test results are normal in about 25% of cases; the transaminases may be slightly raised, but much higher levels suggest other hepatic pathology. Hepatitis viral serology, ultrasonography of the gallbladder to exclude stones, and an autoantibody screen (particularly mitochondrial antibodies for primary biliary cirrhosis) should be performed in all cases as these examine valid differential diagnoses. If clinically indicated, thyroid function tests are also pertinent, and an ultrasound scan to monitor fetal growth should be performed (**Q2**). In this case, these supplementary investigations were normal.

ICP is an idiopathic condition which begins in the second or third trimesters of pregnancy and resolves after delivery. It is thought to result from a genetic predisposition to cholestasis and some data suggest an autosomal dominant inheritance. The biliary obstruction is probably related to changes in the canaliculi induced by altered oestrogen metabolism, which produces an increase in circulating bile salts (**Q3**). The incidence is highly variable, probably reflecting genetic and perhaps geographical or environmental factors. An incidence of approximately 1 per 1000 pregnancies in the UK is exceeded by up to 20-fold, with incidences of over 2% reported in Sweden and among the Araucanian Indians of Chile (**Q4**).

For the mother, ICP is not a life-threatening condition, although the pruritus causes marked discomfort. It carries a 10–20% risk of placental abruption, largely due to hypoprothrombinaemia from vitamin K malabsorption (Shaw *et al*, 1982). Maternal nutritional status may be impaired by steatorrhoea and ICP carries an appreciable risk of present or later cholelithiasis (Shaw *et al*, 1982). Fetal risks for prematurity, intrapartum fetal distress, meconium staining of the amniotic fluid, and stillbirth are all increased, and may be related to the severity of the syndrome. The specific aetiology of the fetal compromise is unknown but may be related to placental insufficiency secondary to impaired hepatic function (such as maternal fat malabsorption) (**Q5: true = A, B, C, D, E**).

Treatment of pruritus in ICP is symptomatic and is rarely satisfactory. Cholestyramine is a resin used to bind the bile acids in the gut. It is the increase in the level of serum bile acids that causes the intense pruritus. However, whilst cholestyramine therapy is theoretically attractive, it is usually unsuccessful. If cholestyramine is used, vitamin K supplements are recommended. Antihistamines may provide slumber and a brief respite. Cool baths, oatmeal baths and bicarbonate washes may help mild cases. Skin emollients are sometimes helpful. Phenol 0.5–1% in aqueous cream, with or without menthol 0.5–1%, may provide local relief. Phenobarbitone, to induce hepatic secretion of bile salts, has not been shown to be effective in controlled trials. Hydroxyethylrutosides, which have been used in primary biliary cirrhosis to reduce bile leakage from dermal capillaries, may be of value and merit further study. Finally, suberythemal doses of ultraviolet B radiation three times weekly can be safe and effective (**Q6**).

When monitoring fetal growth, the abdominal circumference (AC) is the single most effective measurement. The most accurate AC is the smallest one obtained between fetal respirations at the level of the hepatic vein, as the smallest perimeter will be that closest to the plane perpendicular to the spine. The terms intrauterine growth restriction (IUGR) and small for gestational age (SGA) are not synonymous, but are different clinical entities. IUGR implies a failure to achieve genetic growth potential through lack of nutritional support during intrauterine life. Just as a fetus with an AC above the 10th centile may be growth retarded, a fetus with an AC below the 5th centile may not have IUGR. The head circumference is not subject to the extrinsic variability of the biparietal diameter – the shape of the cranium is readily altered by external forces. In addition a technically adequate biparietal diameter cannot be measured if the fetal head is in a direct anterior–posterior position (**Q7: true = A; false = B, C, D**).

Parameters of biophysical profile scoring include fetal breathing movements, gross body/limb movements, fetal tone and posture, fetal heart rate reactivity and amniotic fluid volume estimation (ultrasound estimation of fetal growth and ultrasound estimation of fetal growth are not included). For each parameter, a score of 2 is given, if the criteria for normal behaviour are met. Amniotic fluid volume has emerged as the most important variable, and the finding of oligohydramnios constitutes an abnormal assessment, even if the other parameters are normal. Because of intrinsic cyclicity, fetal breathing movements are, indeed, the parameter most likely to be absent in an otherwise normal profile. In large studies, the negative predictive value (normal score, still healthy at 7 days) is over 99.9%, and less than 1% of fetuses score below 6/10 (Harman *et al*, 1995). A score of 4/10 indicates that acute fetal asphyxia is likely and is an indication for delivery (**Q8: true = A, C, E, F, G; false = B, D**).

The recurrence rate in future pregnancies is approximately 50% (Shaw *et al*, 1982). In women who have had ICP, administration of the combined oral contraceptive pill has been reported to precipitate a recurrence. However, most of these reports quote high steroid doses. Modern combined pills may be considered in a patient who has suffered ICP, provided liver enzymes are checked regularly, and the medication is stopped at the first complaint of pruritus (**Q9**).

REFERENCES

Harman CR, Menticoglou SM, Manning FA, Albar H, Morrison I. Prenatal fetal monitoring: abnormalities of fetal behaviour. In: James DK, Steer PJ, Weiner CP, Gonik B (eds) *High Risk Pregnancy*, pp. 693–734. London: WB Saunders, 1995.

Shaw D, Frohlich J, Wittmann BA, Willms M. A prospective study of 18 patients with cholestasis of pregnancy. *Am J Obstet Gynecol* 1982; **142**: 621–625.

FACTS YOU SHOULD HAVE LEARNT . . .

- ▶ The differential diagnosis of pruritus in pregnancy
- ▶ The characteristic features of intrahepatic cholestasis of pregnancy
- ▶ The management of intrahepatic cholestasis of pregnancy
- ▶ The parameters of the biophysical profile score

CASE 17

Rhesus isoimmunization

A 22-year-old married Caucasian woman was referred to the antenatal booking clinic in her first pregnancy. She was a non-smoker and had no significant past medical or family history. At 10 weeks' gestation her weight was 90 kg, blood pressure was 130/70 mmHg and there were no abnormalities on physical examination. Her blood group was O rhesus negative with no detected red cell antibodies; the rubella antibody titre indicated immunity and the α-fetoprotein estimation at 16 weeks' gestation was normal. An anomaly scan at 20 weeks' gestation was normal and antenatal care was organized with the primary care community team.

> **Q1:** List the variety of antibodies that can be usefully measured in obstetrics and the situation in which you might want to measure them in the patient's serum.

> **Q2:** What are the UK guidelines for screening for the detection of red cell antibodies and for postnatal prophylaxis in this case?

> **Q3:** What is your recommended routine red cell antibody detection screening programme for rhesus-positive women?

The patient's pregnancy progressed normally without complication until 26 weeks' gestation when the routine red cell antibody screen detected an anti-D antibody in the mother's serum at a level of less than $1\,\mathrm{IU\,l^{-1}}$.

> **Q4:** Which of the following statements regarding her management are correct?
>
> A: The anti-D levels are insignificant and can be ignored.
>
> B: This result could be caused by the administration of anti-D immunoglobulin.
>
> C: The patient's anti-D serum levels should be quantified every 2 weeks.
>
> D: The father's blood group and genotype should be determined.
>
> E: A Kleihauer test should be performed and, if positive, 500 IU anti-D immunoglobulin should be administered to the mother by deep intramuscular injection.

The patient did not give any history of vaginal bleeding or abdominal pain but did remember falling down a few stairs at her home a few weeks beforehand. She had not had anti-D immunoglobulin administered during the pregnancy.

A repeat level 2 weeks later revealed the same level of anti-D antibody in the serum. Her husband's blood group was O rhesus positive with a genotype of *CDe/CDe*.

Q5: Which of the following statements are correct?
  A: All children from this man will be rhesus positive.
  B: Anti-D antibody class is immunoglobulin (Ig) M, which will freely cross the placenta.
  C: Anti-D immunoglobulin administration after the fall may have prevented isoimmunization in this patient.
  D: A rising level of anti-D antibody would indicate increasing risk of fetal red cell haemolysis.

Two weeks later, the serum anti-D antibody level had risen to 3 $IU l^{-1}$. At 34 weeks' gestation the anti-D antibody level had risen to 42 $IU l^{-1}$ and anti-c was also detected in the serum.

Q6: How would you manage the pregnancy from this point?
  A: Administer dexamethasone to the mother to suppress the isoimmunization process?
  B: Deliver the baby immediately as the sudden rise in antibody levels indicates serious fetal compromise and possibly fetal anaemia.
  C: Monitor the fetus closely and perform an amniocentesis to assess the amount of bilirubin in the amniotic fluid.
  D: Discuss with the neonatologists or transfer to a unit with facilities to cope with exchange transfusions.
  E: Deliver the baby immediately if there was any evidence of hydrops fetalis on ultrasound scan.

She was admitted to the antenatal ward for monitoring. Dexamethasone was administered. An ultrasound scan revealed a well grown baby with no evidence of fetal hydrops. Amniocentesis was performed; the amniotic fluid optical density at 450 nm was in region 2A of the Liley prediction chart (suggesting delivery at 35–37 weeks' gestation).

Q7: What arrangements would you make with the blood transfusion laboratory before you delivered this baby?

Q8: What is the Liley prediction chart and what does it predict?

The baby remained active and the cardiotocographs were normal. One week later the anti-D antibody level was 60 $IU l^{-1}$. At 35 weeks' gestation the woman recorded reduced fetal movements and a cardiotocograph had a normal base rate but no accelerations and two small decelerations associated with uterine activity.

An emergency lower segment Caesarean section was organized and a male baby who weighed 2.6 kg was delivered in good condition.

Cord blood results were as follows: haemoglobin 7.8 g dl^{-1}, blood group O rhesus positive, genotype was *CDe/cde*, direct antiglobulin test was positive, bilirubin level was 133 μmol l^{-1}. The baby underwent three exchange transfusions and the maximum bilirubin level was 520 μmol l^{-1}.

Q9: What could the mother's blood group genotype be?

Q10: What are the possible complications for the neonate?

The baby did not develop any respiratory distress and was discharged at 24 days of age, fully breastfed. The baby failed its screening hearing test at 50 dB and paediatric follow-up was arranged.

Q11: What are the implications for this couple in subsequent pregnancies and what would your advice be?

The mother's postoperative course was uncomplicated. The family was seen in the postnatal clinic and the full implications for subsequent pregnancies were discussed.

Q12: Which of the following statements are correct?
A: 125 IU anti-D immunoglobulin will suppress 1 ml of fetal blood in the maternal circulation.
B: 500 IU anti-D immunoglobulin is capable of suppressing at least 99% of all peripartum fetomaternal haemorrhages.
C: Less than 1% of all fetomaternal haemorrhages are greater than 4 ml.
D: A rhesus-positive child will be born to a rhesus-negative mother in 1 in 10 pregnancies in the UK where there are 300 sensitizations per annum.
E: Since the introduction of anti-D immunoprophylaxis in the UK, the number of perinatal deaths due to haemolytic disease of the newborn has fallen by a factor of 1000.
F: Increasing the postpartum dose of anti-D immunoglobulin to 1500 IU in all women will irradicate postpartum rhesus sensitization.
G: In large fetomaternal haemorrhages the maximum amount of anti-D immunoglobulin that can be administered each day is 10 000 IU.

COMMENTARY

Antibodies may be measured in clinical obstetrics in the following situations:

▶ Red cell antibodies.
▶ Indicators of immunity (e.g. rubella, hepatitis, toxoplasmosis).
▶ Indicators of infection (e.g. *Treponema*, herpes, parvovirus).
▶ Indicators of autoimmune disease (e.g. systemic lupus erythematosus, anti-Ro, thyroid disease, antithyroid microsomal antibodies; gestational diabetes, antipancreatic islet cell antibodies).

▶ Antiphospholipid syndromes (e.g. anticardiolipin antibodies).

▶ Thrombocytopenia (e.g. antiplatelet antibodies)   (**Q1**)

In this case, the woman must have screening tests for the development of red cell antibodies at 26–28 and at 36 weeks' gestation. The current UK guidelines for postnatal prophylaxis (National Blood Transfusion Service Immunoglobulin Working Party, 1991) for this woman are:

▶ Determine the rhesus status of the mother and baby (cord blood).

▶ Collect maternal blood for Kleihauer testing.

▶ Administer 500 IU to all rhesus-negative mothers giving birth to rhesus-positive babies (or to babies of unknown rhesus status).

▶ Anti-D immunoglobulin should be given by deep intramuscular injection (deltoid muscle).

▶ Administer dose as soon as possible after delivery and always before 72 hours.

▶ Administer more anti-D immunoglobulin if more than 4 ml of fetal blood is detected in the maternal circulation by Kleihauer testing. (**Q2**)

Rhesus-positive women need be tested only at the booking visit unless they have other red cell antibodies detected or have had previous blood transfusions. These non-Rhesus antibodies may cause problems with haemolytic disease of the newborn and create difficulties with cross-matching blood. Therefore, it would seem good medical practice to send a sample early in labour to alert the transfusion laboratory, to give time to obtain compatible blood. An umbilical cord blood sample should be sent for grouping and direct Coombs' testing as neonatal jaundice may sometimes be encountered (**Q3**).

This woman became sensitized to her baby's blood, with potentially serious implications for the current and subsequent pregnancies. The test results could not be ignored but a history should have been obtained as anti-D immunoglobulin administration can be detected in the maternal serum for up to 6 weeks after administration and its half-life is 20–21 days. It is no use giving anti-D when the damage has already been done (**Q4: true = B, C, D; false = A, E**).

Her husband was homozygous for the D antigen. All his progeny will thus be rhesus positive; indeed, they will all be heterozygous (*D/d*) as the mother must be homozygous for the d antigen (*dd*). IgG can cross the placenta by pinocytosis but IgM class antibodies do not cross the placenta to the fetus. Routine antenatal prophylactic immunization for rhesus-negative women (500 IU at 28 and 34 weeks' gestation) has been shown to reduce the incidence of isoimmunization by 5–7-fold (from 0.9% to 0.16% (Tovey *et al*, 1983)) but has serious resource and cost implications. The advent of specific monoclonal antibodies may resolve the supply problem and anul the potential risk of transmission of viral infections from the polyclonal antibodies from donor plasma, but may increase costs. Rhesus-negative women who suffer abdominal trauma or antepartum haemorrhage should have Kleihauer testing and 500 IU anti-D immunoglobulin. Anti-D antibody quantification does correlate with fetal red cell destruction but will not accurately predict the degree of fetal anaemia. A rough but useful guide for women previously sensitized is: $0-4$ IU l^{-1}, test every second week and deliver at term; $4-10$ IU l^{-1}, deliver at 37 weeks' gestation; $10-15$ IU l^{-1}, first fetal blood at 28 weeks' gestation; > 15 IU l^{-1}, first fetal blood at $20-22$ weeks' gestation or about 10 weeks before the birth gestation of a previously affected infant. Some specialists suggest that cordocentesis is unnecessary with levels of less than 15 IU l^{-1} as most fetuses are not anaemic or only mildly anaemic (Nicholaides and Rodeck, 1992) (**Q5: true = A, C, D, E; false = B**).

Following the rise in titre to 42 IU l^{-1}, assessment of fetal well-being and further assessment of the degree of fetal haemolysis are required. Dexamethasone should be administered to reduce the risks of a preterm delivery. Delivery is indicated if there is any sign of fetal decompensation such as ascites or plural effusions on ultrasound scan, reduced fetal movements and/or cardiotocograph abnormalities including tachycardia, sinusoidal rhythm or unprovoked decelerations. Neonatal and blood transfusion services are essential to treat fetal anaemia and jaundice (**Q6: true = C, D, E; false = A, B**).

Before delivery, the blood transfusion laboratory should be notified and arrangements made to provide irradiated O negative blood for the exchange transfusion of the neonate. The blood must be irradiated to eliminate the possibility of transferring cytomegalovirus to the neonate by the blood. The blood has to be fresh and must be used soon after irradiation (**Q7**).

The Liley prediction chart gives a guide to the obstetrician as to when the baby should be delivered. It is an indirect measure of fetal haemolysis and was devised before the days of cordocentesis and intrauterine transfusion. Cordocentesis is associated with a 1% fetal death rate and thus amniocentesis is a safer option when fetal viability has been established, as in this case. The Liley chart compares the outcome of the pregnancy with the optical density of the amniotic fluid at 450 nm in relation to the gestational age of the pregnancy (**Q8**).

The mother's blood group genotype could be either *cde* or *Cde* (**Q9**).

The possible complications for the neonate were those of preterm delivery and hyperbilirubinaemia, which include deafness and intellectual impairment, and those associated with the exchange blood transfusions, which include viral and bacterial infections, disturbances in electrolytes, cardiac arrhythmias and neonatal death (**Q10**).

The implications for this couple in subsequent pregnancies are that every baby will be affected by this condition, that subsequent pregnancies will have to be monitored carefully and that cordocentesis will probably be necessary at about 24 weeks' gestation (with intrauterine transfusion to attain fetal viability). The complications of these procedures need to be discussed. Artificial insemination with a rhesus-negative donor is a possibility if subsequent pregnancies are unsuccessful (**Q11**).

The introduction of anti-D immunoprophylaxis in the UK in 1961 has resulted in a reduction by a factor of 1000 in the perinatal mortality due to haemolytic disease of the newborn. 125 IU anti-D immunoglobulin will suppress 1 ml of fetal blood in the maternal circulation. Less than 1% of all fetomaternal haemorrhages are more than 4 ml, thus 500 IU anti-D immunoglobulin is capable of suppressing at least 99% of all peripartum fetomaternal haemorrhages. Increasing the postpartum dose of anti-D immunoglobulin does not reduce or irradicate postpartum sensitizations (**Q12: true = A, B, C, D, E, G; false = F**).

REFERENCES

National Blood Transfusion Service Immunoglobulin Working Party. Recommendations for the use of anti-D immunoglobulin. *Prescribers' Journal* 1991; **30**:137–145.

Nicholaides KH, Rodeck CH. Maternal serum anti-D antibody concentration and assessment of rhesus isoimmunisation. *BMJ* 1992; **304**: 1155–1156.

Tovey LAD, Stephenson BJ, Townley A, Taverner J. The Yorkshire antenatal anti-D trial in primigravidae. *Lancet* 1983; **ii**: 244–246.

FACTS YOU SHOULD HAVE LEARNT . . .

▶ **The guidelines for routine screening for the detection of red cell antibodies and routine postnatal prophylaxis**
▶ **The investigation and treatment of pregnancies complicated by haemolytic disease of the newborn**
▶ **Neonatal problems in haemolytic disease of the newborn**

CASE 18

Sickle cell disease

A 17-year-old P0 + 0 woman of African–American origin attended the antenatal booking clinic at 12 weeks' gestation. She gave a history of sickle cell disease (HbSS) that had been diagnosed in the first year of her life. She had had repeated crises requiring hospitalization, the most recent being 3 months before conception. Blood transfusions had been infrequent, with her crises usually treated with hydration, oxygen, analgesics and antibiotics. She had never used any contraception, and had become sexually active (with several different partners) 12 months earlier. She was uncertain of the identity or whereabouts of the father of the pregnancy. Her blood group was A rhesus positive with no red cell antibodies detected.

On examination, she was a slightly built young woman, with a blood pressure of 90/40 mmHg and a pulse of 80 beats per minute. Optic fundoscopy was normal, and she had no leg ulcers. An ultrasound scan was consistent with an 11-week intrauterine gestation.

> **Q1:** **When you counsel the patient, which of the following statements regarding sickle cell disease are accurate?**
> A: Prenatal diagnosis can be obtained after chorionic villus sampling, amniocentesis or cordocentesis.
> B: Haematological analysis of fetal blood samples is the optimal method of prenatal diagnosis.
> C: Maternal mortality rates for women with HbSS in the UK are over 10%.
> D: The perinatal mortality rate in the UK approaches 40% for women with HbSS disease.

The patient did not wish to consider either pregnancy termination or prenatal diagnosis.

> **Q2:** **What investigations would you arrange?**

> **Q3:** **Would you prescribe iron and folate supplementation?**

The haemoglobin level was 8.7 g dl^{-1} and the haematocrit was 24%. Haemoglobin electrophoresis showed 87% HbS, 10% HbF and 3% HbA$_2$. She was seen every 2 weeks in the antenatal clinic as an outpatient until 26 weeks' gestation.

> **Q4:** **Which of the following complications of pregnancy are increased in sickle cell disease?**
> A: Pyelonephritis.
> B: Gestational diabetes.

C: Pre-eclampsia.
D: Intrauterine fetal growth restriction.
E: Polyhydramnios.

At 26 weeks' gestation the patient was admitted for a prophylactic partial exchange transfusion (PPET). She received 5 units of genotypically cross-matched packed red blood cells via PPET. The haemoglobin concentration was 12.3 g dl^{-1} after the transfusion.

Q5: Would you advocate prophylactic partial exchange transfusion? What are the advantages and disadvantages?

The patient had two subsequent admissions during the pregnancy, the first with a urinary tract infection (treated with intravenous ampicillin) and the second with an acute pain crisis (managed with intravenous fluids, antibiotics, warmth, analgesia and a 3-unit blood transfusion). The patient was admitted in spontaneous labour at 38 weeks' gestation.

Q6: In the management of her labour, which of the following would you advise?
A: The fetus should be monitored continuously.
B: Caesarean section is strictly contraindicated.
C: Epidural is to be preferred over spinal anaesthesia.
D: The third stage should be managed actively.

After a labour lasting 11 hours, with epidural anaesthesia, a male infant weighing 3.01 kg was delivered vaginally over an intact perineum. Apgar scores at 1 and 5 minutes were 8 and 10 respectively.

Q7: Will electrophoresis of fetal cord blood accurately predict the prognosis of this patient's child?

Q8: How would you manage the puerperium?

The patient did not breastfeed her child. She was discharged home 6 days after delivery, to return 2 weeks later for contraceptive advice.

Q9: When you are giving contraceptive advice, which of the following methods of contraception are contraindicated?
A: The combined oral contraceptive pill.
B: Injectable progestogens (e.g. Depo-Provera).
C: The intrauterine device.
D: Laparoscopic sterilization.
E: Progestin-only preparations.
F: Barrier contraception.

COMMENTARY

The sickle cell gene is widely distributed around the world and it is estimated that there are about 5000 sufferers of sickle cell disease in the UK. Ideally, the initial presentation should be before conception so that an expert haematological and obstetric opinion can be obtained. Partners should be tested for sickle cell disease or sickle cell trait so that appropriate genetic counselling can be given.

There is wide geographical variation in morbidity and mortality, with a maternal mortality rate in the UK of the order of 1–2% and a perinatal mortality rate of about 5%. Counselling needs to be sensitive, as the mother may be considering terminating a pregnancy for a condition from which she suffers herself. Prenatal diagnosis is achieved by recombinant DNA techniques on small DNA samples obtained by chorionic villus sampling or amniocentesis. This has largely superseded the need for haematological analysis of fetal blood samples. (**Q1: true = A; false = B, C, D**).

Investigations at the booking visit should include haemoglobin estimation, quantitative electrophoresis, blood group and antibodies, liver function tests, serum ferritin, rubella, hepatitis B and C, serology for syphilis, and mid-stream urine microscopy and culture (**Q2**). Folic acid should be prescribed, but biochemical evidence of iron deficiency should be obtained before supplementation as iron stores may have accrued from previous transfusions (**Q3**). During pregnancy, patients with sickle cell disease are at an increased risk of sickle crises, urinary tract infection, pyelonephritis, pneumonia, pre-eclampsia (although this is not a universal finding) and anaemia. Fetal mortality and morbidity often results from exacerbations of maternal disease leading to stillbirth and prematurity. Serial ultrasound scans of fetal growth and well-being should be performed in the third trimester (**Q4: true = A, C, D; false = B, E**).

There is little argument regarding the need for blood transfusion where major complications of sickle cell disease occur. However, the use of PPET is a controversial issue. Some studies have reported no improvement in pregnancy outcome, and possible disadvantages include antibody formation, volume overload, haemochromatosis, increased cost and hospitalization, transmission of infection and psychological dependence (e.g. Miller *et al*, 1981). Other reports have demonstrated reduced numbers of HbS cells, increased HbA cells, suppression of HbS erythropoiesis, decreased perinatal wastage and prematurity, and increased birthweight (e.g. Morrison *et al*, 1991). The only randomized prospective study (of 72 patients) found that the only improved outcome was a reduction in painful crises, and the authors concluded that prophylactic transfusion programmes were not justified (Koshy *et al*, 1988) (**Q5**). A transfusion policy that is often employed is to transfuse when a clear indication is present (severe anaemia $< 6 \, \mathrm{g \, dl^{-1}}$, recurrent crises, multiple pregnancy).

Patients should be kept warm and adequately hydrated in labour, and hypoxia and acidosis should be avoided. The compromised fetal environment results in an increased incidence of fetal distress and Caesarean section. Continuous fetal monitoring should be employed. Regional anaesthesia is preferable as there are risks for general anaesthesia if oxygenation is not maintained. There is a greater risk of hypotension with spinal compared with epidural anaesthesia. The third stage should be managed actively and carefully to minimize blood loss, and transfusion should be used only if necessary (**Q6: true = A, C, D; false = B**).

Fetal cord blood should be taken for electrophoresis, but this should be repeated after 6 months when fetal haemoglobin levels have fallen, as β-chain globin variants will be seen only in the adult haemoglobin (**Q7**).

The puerperium is complicated by infections (chest and urinary tract infections, and endometritis). In addition, death from pulmonary embolism and sickle crises has been reported in the immediate puerperium. Following delivery, patients should be kept warm and hydrated, and prophylactic heparin and antibiotic therapy are sensible precautions (**Q8**).

There is no evidence that patients with sickle cell disease are less fertile than other women, so the need for effective contraception is great. The combined oral contraceptive pill presents (at least) theoretical problems, because oestrogen increases blood coagulability and thus lowers the threshold for crises. Gallbladder disease, another contraindication to the combined pill, is also more common in patients with sickle cell disease. Manufacturers' data sheets list sickle cell disease as a contraindication to the use of the combined contraceptive pill. Nevertheless, combined pill use undoubtedly presents a smaller risk than does pregnancy, and the view that sickle cell disease is only a relative contraindication to use of the combined pill is widely held. Progestin-only contraceptives such as the progestogen-only pill and long-acting intramuscular medroxyprogesterone acetate are good choices. The intrauterine device poses at least theoretical risks of excessive vaginal bleeding, endometritis and tubo-ovarian abscess, with the possibility of provoking sickling crises. Barrier methods of contraception have few side-effects, but the relatively high failure rates make their use of dubious value. Even in an older woman, a laparoscopic sterilization procedure would be contraindicated. Pulmonary aeration is compromised because of the relatively high fixed position of the diaphragm, and a raised $P\text{co}_2$ and lowered pH results from absorption across the peritoneal surface. If patients with sickle cell disease, after achieving a successful pregnancy outcome, opt for permanent sterilization, an interval minilaparotomy procedure (ideally under local anaesthesia) is recommended (**Q9: true = D, perhaps A, C, F; false = B, E**).

REFERENCES

Koshy M, Burd L, Wallace D, Moawad A, Barron J. Prophylactic red-cell transfusions in pregnant patients with sickle cell disease. *N Engl J Med* 1988; **319**: 1447–1452.

Miller JM, Horger EO, Key TC, Walker EM. Management of sickle haemoglobinopathies in pregnant patients. *Am J Obstet Gynecol* 1981; **141**: 237–241.

Morrison JC, Morrison FS, Floyd RC *et al*. Use of continuous flow erythrocytapheresis in pregnant women with sickle cell disease. *J Clin Apheresis* 1991; **6**: 224–229.

FACTS YOU SHOULD HAVE LEARNT . . .

▶ The management of a pregnant patient with sickle cell disease: (i) antepartum, (ii) interpartum, (iii) postpartum
▶ Contraception issues in women with sickle cell disease

CASE 19

Twin pregnancy

A 34-year-old para 0 + 1 Caucasian woman attended the antenatal booking clinic at 13 weeks' gestation. Her previous pregnancy had ended in a spontaneous miscarriage at 6 weeks' gestation. Her past medical history was unremarkable. An ultrasound scan indicated a twin pregnancy, with the crown–rump lengths consistent with her gestational age. A septum was identified, and a single placenta was noted.

QI: **Which of the following statements regarding the incidence of twin pregnancies are correct?**
A: The incidence of twin deliveries in England and Wales is approximately 12.5 per 1000.
B: The worldwide incidence of twin pregnancies varies geographically by up to tenfold.
C: The incidence of dizygotic twinning is relatively constant.
D: The incidence of monozygous twinning is affected by maternal age, parity and ethnic origin.
E: The incidence of twin pregnancies in England and Wales has increased in recent years.

Q2: Which of the following statements regarding the outcomes of twin pregnancies are correct?
A: Perinatal mortality rates in twin pregnancies are fivefold those of singleton pregnancies.
B: Perinatal mortality rates in monochorionic twin pregnancies are five-fold those of dichorionic twin pregnancies.
C: The incidence of small-for-gestational age babies is three times that of singleton pregnancies.
D: The risk of cerebral palsy is eightfold that of singleton pregnancies.
E: The preterm delivery rate in twin pregnancies is approximately 15%.

The patient was rescanned at 15 weeks' gestation after an episode of prolonged heavy vaginal bleeding. An area of reduced echogenicity adjacent to the placenta was found, and was thought to represent a haematoma. Prophylactic iron and folic acid supplementation was commenced. The vaginal bleeding resolved and when the patient attended the antenatal clinic at 19 weeks' gestation, a detailed ultrasound scan was performed. The septum was again noted. Both fetuses were found to be male, and no structural anomalies were seen. A disparity in fetal size was noted; whilst the measurements of one twin were consistent with her gestational age, the biparietal diameter (BPD), head circumference (HC), abdominal circumference (AC) and femur length (FL) of the other twin were equivalent to 17–18 weeks' gestation.

Q3: Has the chorionicity of this pregnancy been established?

Q4: What is the best antenatal method of establishing chorionicity?

Q5: What are the advantages of establishing chorionicity?

The patient remained asymptomatic and reattended the antenatal clinic at 24+ weeks' gestation. An ultrasound scan confirmed that fetal growth of the larger twin remained consistent with her gestational age (BPD: 64 mm, AC 223 mm, approximating to the 50th centile, as illustrated in Figure 1), but those of the smaller twin were below the fifth centile for gestational age (BPD 53 mm, AC 184 mm). The liquor volume around each twin was similar.

Q6: What is the differential diagnosis of the discordant fetal growth?

The differential diagnosis was discussed with the patient in detail. A maternal blood sample was taken for syphilis, parvovirus, cytomegalovirus, coxsackie, herpes simplex and toxoplasmosis serology (this screening was negative). Neither the mother nor her partner wished to contemplate any invasive prenatal testing, and after discussing the different options it was decided to await events. Ultrasonographic assessment of fetal growth was repeated at 28 weeks' gestation. Growth of the larger twin remained on the

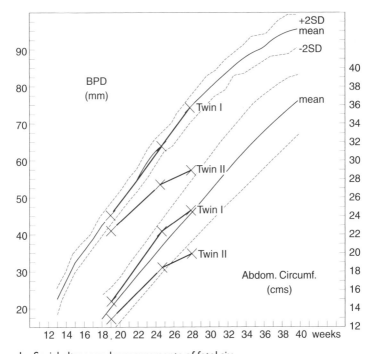

Figure I   Serial ultrasound measurements of fetal six.

50th centile (BPD 74 mm, AC 248 mm), whilst that of the smaller twin was well below the fifth centile (BPD 57 mm, AC 199 mm). The liquor volume around the smaller twin was reduced, with a maximum pool diameter below 1 cm. A biophysical profile was arranged, and was performed the following day (the biophysical profile is discussed in case 16). Unfortunately, no fetal heart was seen in the smaller twin. The biophysical profile score of the larger twin was 10/10.

The patient was admitted to the antenatal ward. She was naturally very anxious and distressed. In an effort to assist the grieving process, she was counselled extensively by the hospital chaplain. Auscultation of the fetal heart rate was performed twice daily, and both the rate and rhythm remained within the normal range. Two intramuscular doses of dexamethasone (12 mg) were administered. One week after the death of the smaller twin, the biophysical profile was repeated; the score was again 10/10. She remained extremely distressed, and after extensive discussion involving the obstetricians, paediatricians and the couple, the decision to perform a Caesarean section at 29+ weeks' gestation was taken.

Q7:   What are the advantages and disadvantages of delivering the surviving twin at this gestation?

A lower segment Caesarean section was performed under spinal anaesthesia (a maternal clotting screen was normal). The lie of both twins was longitudinal, with cephalic presentations. Twin I was delivered in good condition to the awaiting paediatrician. Twin I breathed spontaneously with Apgar scores of 8 at 1 minute, and 10 at 5 minutes. The birthweight of twin I was 1.31 kg. Twin II was a macerated stillbirth weighing 0.64 kg. No dysmorphic features were seen.

Q8:   What investigations would you perform to establish the cause of the intrauterine fetal death?

All investigations were unremarkable, although it was not possible to obtain a karyotypic analysis of the macerated twin. The post-mortem examination revealed no abnormalities apart from gross growth restriction. The postdelivery progress of both mother and baby was excellent, and the surviving twin was discharged home 7 weeks after delivery.

COMMENTARY

The true incidence of twinning is impossible to determine as early *in utero* losses are unknown. However, the Registrar General's 1992 review shows that the incidence of twin deliveries was 12 per 1000 in England and Wales. This rate has increased from 10 per 1000 over recent years owing to the increased availability of assisted conception rates. There is a marked geographical variation in the incidence of twin deliveries, with rates as high as 52 per 1000 in Ghana and as low as 5 per 1000 in Taiwan. The incidence of monozygous twinning is relatively constant at 4 per 1000, and it is the incidence of dizygous twinning that varies with maternal age, parity, ethnic origin and the use of assisted reproductive techniques (**Q1: true = A, B, E; false = C, D**).

The rate of stillbirth in multiple pregnancies is approximately 14 per 1000, compared with 4 per 1000 in singleton pregnancies, and the early neonatal death rate is 25 per 1000 compared with 3 per 1000 (England and Wales, 1992). The factors responsible for the increased pregnancy loss in twin pregnancies include increased incidence of preterm delivery (rates vary between populations from 30% to 50%), intrauterine growth restriction (the incidence of small-for-gestational age babies, defined as below the 10th centile, varies from about 25% to 33%), malpresentation and congenital malformations (major congenital abnormalities are increased by about twofold). Perinatal morbidity and mortality is threefold to fivefold higher in monochorionic than in dichorionic pregnancies. The relative increase in risk in monochorionic compared with dichorionic twin pregnancies approximates to that of twin compared with singleton pregnancies. The risk of cerebral palsy is increased by eightfold in twin pregnancies. Much of the increased mortality and morbidity in twin pregnancies is due to the presence of vascular anastamoses which are implicated in the twin–twin transfusion syndrome and the co-twin sequelae after the intrauterine death of one twin (**Q2: true = A, B, C, D; false = E**).

Prenatal determination of chorionicity is based on the use of ultrasonography to identify fetal sex, the number of placental masses and the inter-twin membrane thickness (Winn et al, 1989). Fetal sexing can be performed on the 18–20-week detailed scan. The accuracy is high provided that visualization of female external genitalia is used as the criterion for female sex rather than the non-visualization of male genitalia. Separate placental masses indicate dichorionicity and discordant external genitalia indicate dizygosity and therefore dichorionicity. Most twins are of like sex and separate placental masses often lie adjacent to each other. In this case, with concordant genitalia and a single placental mass, monochorionic placentation is only a possibility, and the chorionicity has not been established (**Q3**).

The optimal gestation to assess the inter-twin septum is in the first trimester, before 11 weeks' gestation. Dichorionic twins have thicker membranes (the dividing membrane is two layers of chorion and two of amnion) than monochorionic twins (the dividing membrane is two layers of amnion). The chorion in the septum is thicker in early pregnancy before the chorion laeve regresses (Kurtz et al, 1992). Moreover, until the amnion fuses with the chorion late in the first trimester, the constituent layers of the septum can be seen ultrasonographically. Another method of characterizing chorionicity involves the appearance of the septum at its origin from the placenta. A tongue of placental tissue is seen on ultrasound scans, within the base of dichorionic membranes, and has been termed the 'twin peak' or 'lambda' sign. It is thought to represent incomplete regression of the chorion laeve at its junction with the chorion frondosum (Kurtz *et al*, 1992) **(Q4).**

Determination of chorionicity should be performed routinely in multiple pregnancies in all obstetric units. A diagnosis of a monochorionic twin pregnancy places the pregnancy in a high-risk group for several reasons. Firstly, the pregnancy must be dizygous, and thus at an increased risk of congenital abnormality in each pregnancy, with a fourfold increased risk of congenital heart defects in each pregnancy. Secondly, there are implications for prenatal diagnosis, both in the methods of investigation and the interpretation of results. However, the most important reason relates to the presence of vascular anastamoses within the chorionic plate, which may allow twin–twin transfusions to occur. The incidence of twin–twin transfusion syndrome is approximately 10% of all pregnancies. Acute severe twin–twin transfusion syndrome occurs in about 1% of monochorionic gestations. Early confirmation of chorionicity allows increased surveillance of monochorionic pregnancies and hence detection of the potential complications as soon as possible **(Q5).**

As the chorionicity has not been established in this case, the differential diagnosis of the discordant fetal growth must include twin–twin transfusion syndrome. Twin–twin transfusion syndrome involves the transfusion of blood from one twin to the other. Once an unequal anastomosis is established, the donor twin becomes anaemic, hypovolaemic, oligohydramniotic and poorly grown. In contrast, the recipient becomes polycythaemic, hypervolaemic and polyuric, and polyhydramnios develops. The mortality rate for discordant twins presenting at 18–26 weeks' gestation is high, ranging from 80% to 100%. There was no disparity in the liquor volumes around the twins, as would have been anticipated in twin–twin transfusion. Therapeutic amnioreduction is probably the only effective treatment for this complication of monochorionic twin pregnancies, and was clearly not indicated in a case without any liquor volume disparity. The fetal growth restriction of the smaller twin was symmetrical, suggesting a karyotypic abnormality or a fetal infection, rather than a placental cause **(Q6).**

After the death of the smaller twin, the decision to deliver the surviving twin was difficult, and the appropriateness of the decision made is equivocal. The decision was made more difficult by the earlier failure to determine chorionicity. When a single intrauterine death occurs in a monochorionic gestation, the incidence of necrotic neurological and renal lesions is about 25%, with a similar 25% risk of intrauterine death in the initially healthy co-twin. The mechanism of this co-twin compromise is unclear, but it is thought that episodes of haemodynamic imbalance cause periods of hypotension, resulting in ischaemia. In contrast, when a single intrauterine death occurs in a dichorionic pregnancy, these acute risks do not pertain. However, if the pathological condition that resulted in the death of one twin can be identified and persists, delivery may still be indicated. The risks of delivery must be balanced with those of prematurity. The management of this case took place within a regional neonatal referral centre. The local figures for survival of babies delivered at 29+ weeks' gestation approximated to 90% (**Q7**).

Investigation of the cause of the death of growth-restricted twin must include determination of the karyotype. The karyotype should be determined in most fetuses even in the apparent absence of structural malformations, because the usual dysmorphic features may be obscured by post-mortem changes. In contrast to fetal fascia or subcutaneous tissue, amniocytes can be cultured after fetal demise. The placenta is an alternative site for obtaining material for karyotype. Photographs should be made, for both medical records and the parents. The fetal organ cavities should be cultured for both bacteria and viruses, and permission for a post-mortem examination should be sought. Additional maternal blood tests that are routinely performed in intrauterine fetal deaths include glycosylated haemoglobin, Kleihauer test, and detection of anticardiolipin, antinuclear antibodies and lupus anticoagulant (**Q8**).

REFERENCES

Kurtz AB, Wapner RJ, Mata J, Johnson A, Morgan P. Twin pregnancies: accuracy of first trimester abdominal US in predicting chorionicity and amnionicity. *Radiology* 1992; **185**: 759–762.

Winn HN, Gabrielli S, Reece EA, Roberts JA, Salafia C, Hobbins JC. Ultrasonic criteria for the prenatal diagnosis of placental chorionicity in twin gestations. *Am J Obstet Gynecol* 1989; **161**: 1540–1542.

FACTS YOU SHOULD HAVE LEARNT . . .

- The incidence and complications of twin pregnancies
- The method used to determine chorionicity
- The importance of the determination of chorionicity
- The differential diagnosis of discordant fetal growth in a twin pregnancy
- The management after intrauterine fetal death of one fetus in a twin pregnancy

CASE 20

Pre-eclampsia

A 25-year-old P 1+0 Caucasian woman presented to the antenatal booking clinic at 11 weeks' gestation. Four years previously she had undergone an emergency Caesarean section delivery of a male infant weighing 0.97 kg at 32 weeks' gestation. The previous pregnancy had been complicated by intrauterine growth restriction (IUGR) and fulminating pre-eclampsia. There was no relevant past medical history (she was a non-smoker), but her mother had also suffered 'toxaemia' in one of her pregnancies. General examination, including urine analysis, was unremarkable; her weight was 76.8 kg and blood pressure was 110/65 mmHg. An ultrasound scan was consistent with an 11-week intrauterine gestation.

The patient was anxious to know whether she was likely to suffer a recurrence of pre-eclampsia, and mentioned that her general practitioner had discussed 'aspirin treatment' with her.

QI: **Which of the following statements regarding the likelihood of pre-eclampsia (relative to the general pregnant population) are correct?**
A: The risk is minimal, as she is no longer nulliparous.
B: The risk is significantly increased, because of the family history of 'toxaemia'.
C: The risk is significantly increased, as she is Caucasian.
D: The risk is significantly increased, owing to her age.

Q2: **Which of the following statements concerning the use of low-dose aspirin are correct?**
A: There is good evidence to support the use of low-dose aspirin prophylaxis in patients who have had pre-eclampsia in previous pregnancies.
B: The dose of aspirin for pre-eclampsia prophylaxis is 500 mg per day.
C: Due to a well-documented risk of teratogenesis, aspirin should not be used in early pregnancy.
D: Pre-eclampsia prophylaxis is most effective when started before 16 weeks' gestation.
E: Aspirin inhibits the cyclo-oxygenase enzyme and inhibits thromboxane production.

Q3: **Are you aware of any techniques that are useful and reliable screening tests for predicting the development of pre-eclampsia?**

A detailed ultrasound scan at 18 weeks' gestation revealed no abnormality, and the pregnancy was uncomplicated until 25 weeks' gestation when the patient presented to her community midwife with a 1-day history of generalized swelling and a headache. Her blood pressure was 140/90 mmHg and on dipstick testing of the urine, protein+++ was revealed. The on-call obstetric registrar at the local teaching hospital was contacted and an emergency admission was arranged.

Q4: Which of the following criteria have to be met in order to diagnose pre-eclampsia?

A: Oedema must be present.

B: Proteinuria must be greater than I g per litre.

C: There must be no evidence of renal dysfunction.

D: Diastolic blood pressure must be greater than 90 mmHg.

On admission, the patient's headache had resolved. Generalized oedema, involving the upper and lower limbs, and face, was noted. There was no epigastric tenderness or hyperreflexia detected. The blood pressure was again noted as 140/90 mmHg and proteinuria +++ was found.

Q5: Which of the following investigations are appropriate?

A: Plasma urate estimation.

B: Platelet count.

C: 24-hour estimation of urinary protein.

D: Plasma renin concentration.

E: Measurement of circulating levels of tumour necrosis factor (TNF) α.

F: Liver function tests.

The results of initial biochemical and haematological investigations were within normal limits. An ultrasound scan was performed, and indicated asymmetrical IUGR, with the abdominal circumference measurements below the fifth centile for gestational age, and the head circumference and biparietal diameters approximating to the 50th centile. Umbilical artery Doppler studies indicated reversed end-diastolic blood flow.

She remained an inpatient, with the blood pressure consistently measured at 140/90 mmHg, and biochemical and haematological investigations remained within normal limits. On the third day following admission, a 24-hour urine collection was reported as containing 3.95 g protein. On the fifth day, blood pressure recordings were persistently raised (180/95 mmHg) and oral labetalol therapy (100 mg three times daily) was commenced. Two doses of dexamethasone (12 mg) were administered intramuscularly, 12 hours apart.

Q6: Would you have prescribed labetalol?

Q7: Would you have prescribed dexamethasone?

The patient's blood pressure was stable (140/85 mmHg) on labetalol therapy, and on the seventh day after admission a 24-hour urine collection was found to contain 5.25 g protein. On the ninth day, the platelet count had fallen to 80×10^9 l^{-1} (other biochemical and haematological investigations remained within normal limits), and the blood pressure was persistently raised at 190/110 mmHg despite labetalol therapy. The decision to stabilize her condition and then deliver the baby was taken.

The blood pressure was controlled with an infusion of 50 mg hydralazine in 50 ml normal saline at 1–5 mg per hour, aiming to achieve blood pressure recordings below 160/90–100 mmHg. An initial 4-g bolus dose of magnesium sulphate was infused over 20 minutes; the infusion continued at 4.5 g per hour, reducing to 3 g per hour. Urine output remained above 40 ml per hour.

Q8: Would you have used an alternative anticonvulsant agent?

Q9: Which of the following statements concerning the use of magnesium sulphate are correct?
   A. Serum magnesium levels should remain between 20 and 25 mmol l^{-1}
   B. Respiratory depression caused by hypermagnesaemia should be reversed by 1 ml of 1:10 000 adrenaline.
   C. The absence of deep tendon reflexes should lead you to check magnesium levels and consider reducing the infusion.
   D. Signs of hypomagnesaemia include flushing, sweating and hypotension.

A male infant weighing 540 g was delivered by classical Caesarean section, and the patient's clinical condition improved rapidly following delivery. Magnesium sulphate and hydralazine infusions were discontinued 24 hours after delivery; urine output remained excellent, and she had no postoperative complications. When reviewed six weeks after delivery, she was normotensive (110/70 mmHg) and had no proteinuria. Biochemical assessments of liver and renal function remained within normal limits.

Unfortunately, all efforts to treat the baby were unsuccessful. At delivery he had a heart rate of 60 beats per minute and was intubated and ventilated. However, it was difficult to achieve adequate ventilation, and severe hyaline membrane disease was confirmed on chest radiography; there was no response to two doses of surfactant. He was jaundiced from day 2, and required phototherapy. He became hypotensive and a dopamine infusion was instigated. On day 2 his abdomen became distended and necrotizing enterocolitis was diagnosed after abdominal radiography; total parenteral nutrition was commenced. On day 5, grade II-III intraventricular haemorrhages were found on ultrasound scan. After discussion with his parents, intensive care was withdrawn and he died after 6 days of life.

COMMENTARY

Pre-eclampsia is principally a disease of nulliparous women, and a diagnosis of pre-eclampsia in a multiparous woman whose previous pregnancies have been uncomplicated should be treated with suspicion.

However, the incidence of pre-eclampsia in a woman whose previous pregnancy has been complicated by pre-eclampsia is approximately 25%. A family history of pre-eclampsia is associated with a threefold increase in the incidence of pre-eclampsia. The risk of developing pre-eclampsia is not increased by either age or Caucasian origin. Pre-eclampsia is most common in women below 15 years or above 35 years of age, and in those of African origin (**Q1: true = B; false = A, C, D**).

Aspirin acetylates the active site of the cyclo-oxygenase enzyme and thus inhibits eicosanoid production. Platelets, which predominantly produce the vasoconstrictor thromboxane, lack nuclei and cannot resynthesize the enzyme. Endothelial cells have the capacity to synthesize new enzymes and thus can produce the vasodilator prostacyclin when aspirin is removed from the system. The net effect is a reduction in the thromboxane : prostacyclin ratio, and can be achieved by a dose of as little as 37.5 mg per day (although 75 mg tablets are the only commercially available preparations). Although several small studies have suggested that low-dose aspirin might be effective in preventing pre-eclampsia, a number of large prospective randomized trials (the largest of which was the CLASP study, 1994) have failed to show any significant effect. Aspirin appears to be free of teratogenic effects. There is some evidence from subanalysis of the CLASP study that aspirin, if taken before 16 weeks' gestation, reduces the incidence of early-onset pre-eclampsia (**Q2: true = D, E; false = A, B, C**).

Over 100 clinical, physiological and biochemical tests have been suggested in the prediction of pre-eclampsia, in keeping with the legion of possible aetiological factors that have been proposed. Apart from a detailed family and past medical history, there is no practical, acceptable and reliable screening test for the development of pre-eclampsia that has been thoroughly tried and tested. There are tests that are potentially useful (including plasma fibronectin estimation and colour flow Doppler imaging of uterine arteries), but in the absence of useful prophylactic therapy, the possible applications are limited (**Q3**).

There are many different definitions and classifications of pregnancy-induced hypertension and pre-eclampsia. Arguably the best of these are those of the International Society for the Study of Hypertension in Pregnancy: pregnancy-induced hypertension is defined as a diastolic blood pressure of 90 mmHg or greater, on two consecutive recordings at least 4 hours apart, occurring in a previously normotensive woman after the 20th week of pregnancy; pre-eclampsia is defined as pregnancy-induced hypertension with the addition of significant proteinuria (greater than 300 mg per 24 hours in the absence of a urinary tract infection). One of the problems of the definition used by the American College of Obstetricians and Gynecologists is that the criteria for hypertension (an increase in diastolic blood pressure of at least 15 mmHg) is met at some stage in the pregnancies of approximately 25% of women. Oedema is not included in the definition of pre-eclampsia. Oedema is present in 80% of pregnancies and, indeed, is associated with a favourable prognosis.

However, the presence of generalized oedema, involving the upper limbs and face, is a useful sign. Renal dysfunction does not preclude the diagnosis (**Q4: true = D; false = A, B, C**).

Uric acid is excreted primarily through the renal tubules, and plasma urate estimations are a sensitive indicator of renal function and renal blood flow. Both plasma urate estimation and the platelet count (which falls as disseminated intravascular coagulation occurs) are useful markers of the disease process. Proteinuria is best estimated as a 24-hour loss, and whenever possible should be quantified to confirm the diagnosis (although with +++ on dipstick testing, it is very unlikely that this patient's proteinuria had nˊt attained significant levels). Plasma levels of renin and TNF-α are increased in pre-eclampsia, but these measurements are not of value in managing the case. Abnormal liver function test results (particularly transaminase estimation) are indicative of severe disease (**Q5: true=A, B, C, F; false = D, E**).

It is difficult to assess whether the labetolol therapy was beneficial. Antihypertensive drugs lower blood pressure – they should not be expected to do anything else, and will not affect the underlying disease process. The aim of therapy is to reduce the risk to the mother by preventing progressive vascular damage and cerebral vascular accident. By lowering the perceived risk it may be possible to allow the pregnancy to continue to the benefit of the fetus by increasing maturity. Randomized controlled comparisons between labetalol (an alpha- and beta-blocker) and placebo have failed to demonstrate any beneficial effect. However, all the randomized studies of the effects of treating of pre-eclampsia with antihypertensive medication have been too small to provide reliable information on safety or efficacy, even when considered together using meta-analysis. In view of the likely problems of prematurity consequent upon delivery at such an early gestation, the decision to prescribe labetalol does not seem unreasonable (**Q6**). Although her gestational age was outside that of many studies of the effects of corticosteroid administration, the benefits of such therapy on fetal lung maturity are so well established that prescribing dexamethasone was in accord with standard practice. Two contradictory findings are particularly pertinent. One is the report (in one of three studies to have focused on patients with pre-eclampsia) that corticosteroid administration predisposes to fetal death in women with pre-eclampsia; the other is the intriguing finding of an improvement in the clinical condition of women with early-onset severe pre-eclampsia following dexamethasone administration (**Q7**).

Hydralazine is the antihypertensive agent most commonly used in the UK in the acute management of hypertension in pregnancy, although intravenous labetalol infusion is a good alternative. Although the most commonly used anticonvulsant agent in the UK is diazepam, the use of magnesium sulphate to prevent convulsions is routine in North America. In comparisons of magnesium sulphate and diazepam, when used to prevent further convulsions after an eclamptic fit, magnesium sulphate has been shown to be both safe and more effective. Phenytoin administration has also been advocated, but, although effective in the treatment of epilepsy, it is of dubious benefit in preventing eclampsia. There are those who do not use anticonvulsant therapy in patients who have not had seizures, arguing that such treatment has not been subjected to randomized controlled trials. Whilst this is true, the sample size that such a study would require to attain sufficient power is probably prohibitive, particularly in view of the excellent results obtained by protagonists of the use of magnesium sulphate (Sibai, 1990) (**Q8**).

The therapeutic range of magnesium is 2–2.5 mmol l^{-1}. Deep tendon reflexes are depressed at about 4 mmol l^{-1} and may be lost at 5 mmol l^{-1}, at which level respiratory paralysis may occur. If the deep tendon reflexes are absent, the magnesium infusion must be stopped. Magnesium concentrations above 6 mmol l^{-1} may be fatal. Signs of hypermagnesaemia include: flushing, sweating, hypotension, depression of reflexes, flaccid paralysis, hypothermia, circulatory collapse and depression of cardiac and central nervous system function. Respiratory depression caused by hypermagnesaemia should be reversed by the intravenous administration of 10–20 ml 10% calcium gluconate (**Q9: true = D; false = A, B, C**). You must be familiar with the pre-eclampsia protocol of your unit.

REFERENCES

CLASP (Collaborative Low Dose Aspirin Study in Pregnancy) Collaborative Group. CLASP: a randomised trial of low-dose aspirin for the prevention and treatment of pre-eclampsia among 9364 pregnant women. *Lancet* 1994; **343**: 619–629.

Sibai BM. Magnesium sulfate is the ideal convulsant in preeclampsia–eclampsia. *Am J Obstet Gynecol* 1990; **162**: 1141–1145.

FACTS YOU SHOULD HAVE LEARNT . . .

- ▶ The risk factors for pre-eclampsia
- ▶ The evidence for prophylaxis of pre-eclampsia using low-dose aspirin
- ▶ The diagnostic criteria for pre-eclampsia
- ▶ The appropriate investigations in pre-eclampsia
- ▶ The treatment options in pre-eclampsia

CASE 21

Preterm rupture of membranes

A 30-year-old P1 + 1 Caucasian woman presented to the antenatal booking clinic at 12 weeks' gestation. Her previous pregnancy had been complicated by preterm rupture of membranes at 33 weeks' gestation. Although her daughter had been admitted to the special care baby unit for 4 weeks, she was now an entirely normal 3-year-old child. There was no other relevant past medical history (the patient was a smoker). General examination was unremarkable. An ultrasound scan was consistent with a 12-week intrauterine gestation.

The patient was anxious to know whether she was likely to suffer a recurrence of preterm rupture of membranes, and whether she could do anything to prevent such a recurrence.

Q1:   How would you have addressed her anxieties?

A routine detailed ultrasound scan at 20 weeks' gestation was unremarkable.

At 25 weeks' gestation she was admitted to the labour ward with a good history of her membranes having ruptured 3 hours before admission. She had not noted any uterine activity. On examination the blood pressure was 135/65 mmHg, temperature was 37.0°C, and the pulse rate was 95 beats per minute (bpm). No contractions were observed, and the fetal heart rate was approximately 140 bpm. An aseptic speculum examination was performed and clear fluid was seen in the vagina. A high vaginal swab was taken.

Q2:   When the history of rupture of membranes is equivocal, which of the following investigations are helpful?
A: Nitrazine pH sticks.
B: Ultrasonographic estimation of amniotic fluid.
C: Fetal fibronectin estimation.
D: Intra-amniotic injection of dye.

Q3:   At what stage of gestational development can a fetus survive outside the uterus?

Q4:   In preterm rupture of membranes, which of the following interventions result in a demonstrable reduction in perinatal mortality?
A: Corticosteroid administration.
B: β-Mimetic tocolytic therapy.
C: Antibiotic administration.
D: Hospitalization.
E: Corticosteroid administration and induction of labour.

After 4 hours of observation on the labour ward, during which time the clinical signs were largely unchanged, the patient was transferred to the antenatal ward. Intramuscular dexamethasone was administered, and she was entered into the ORACLE study (a randomized placebo-controlled trial of the use of antibiotics in premature labour). An ultrasound scan the following day revealed marked oligohydramnios (with a maximal pool depth of 1 cm), measurements of fetal size that were consistent with gestational age, and a flexed breech presentation.

Q5: What forms of monitoring would you instigate?

Microbiological culture of the vaginal swab did not indicate any infection. Over the next 6 days on the antenatal ward, the patient continued to note clear fluid draining vaginally, but was otherwise asymptomatic, and clinical signs were unremarkable.

Q6: Which of the following statements concerning preterm rupture of membranes are correct?
A: Delivery occurs within 1 week of preterm premature rupture of membranes in about 50% of cases.
B: The incidence of chorioamnionitis is approximately 30%.
C: The incidence of neonatal sepsis approximates to that of chorioamnionitis.
D: The chance of infection is greatest at early gestational ages.
E: The chance of infection is greatest when the latent period is long.

On the seventh day following admission, she noted the onset of regular, painful uterine contractions. She had remained apyrexial. On vaginal examination, the cervix was noted to be 4 cm dilated.

Q7: How would you deliver the baby?

A female infant weighing 1.2 kg was delivered by classical Caesarean section under general anaesthesia.

Q8: What are the indications for classical Caesarean section?

Q9: Which of the following statements concerning classical Caesarean section are correct?
A: There is no dissection of the bladder.
B: The incidence of postoperative infection is increased relative to that of a lower segment Caesarean section.
C: A subsequent trial of labour is contraindicated.
D: Encroachment into the active upper segment is unusual.

Q10: With regard to women delivering after preterm rupture of membranes, what postnatal complications are particularly important?

The postnatal course was largely uncomplicated. There was no evidence of neonatal infection or respiratory distress syndrome; the major problem was neonatal jaundice which responded well to phototherapy. Six months after delivery, no significant infant morbidity was evident.

COMMENTARY

Preterm rupture of membranes is defined as rupture of the fetal membranes with a latent period before the onset of spontaneous uterine activity, at a gestation of less than 37 completed weeks. The incidence approximates to 2% of all pregnancies.

The recurrence rate for preterm rupture of membranes is between 20% and 30%. Smoking is an independent risk factor and there is some evidence that cessation of smoking reduces the incidence of this complication. The importance of maternal vaginal colonization of potentially pathogenic microorganisms in the aetiology of premature rupture of membranes is uncertain. The benefits of vaginal cultures and prophylactic antimicrobial therapy have not been proven. Prophylactic treatment of the sexual partner is even more contentious, whilst restriction of sexual activity during pregnancy cannot be justified on current evidence (**Q1**).

If a history is suggestive of premature rupture of membranes, an aseptic vaginal speculum examination should be performed. Visualization of liquor draining through the cervix is the best method for confirming the diagnosis. Use of nitrazine sticks is dependent on the alkaline liquor turning the pH indicator black. However, vaginal infection or urine can have a similar effect on pH, and the false-positive rate using the sticks is about 25%. Ultrasonographic diagnosis of polyhydramnios is often possible only after a large fluid loss which is clinically obvious. Recent evidence suggests that fetal fibronectin estimation may be an effective method of predicting premature labour (Lockwood, 1995), and it may prove an effective method of diagnosing premature rupture of membranes. The invasive intra-amniotic injection of dyes is not without hazard, and is not widely practised (**Q2: true = possibly C; false = A, B, D**).

The growing perception that technology is pushing back the frontiers of fetal viability led Governor Cuomo of New York to establish a task force to examine the question of at what stage can a fetus survive *ex utero* (Committee on Fetal Extrauterine Survivability, 1988). The task force identified three organ systems as essential to fetal survival: brain, kidneys and lungs. Of these, lung development was considered the most critical. It was concluded that gas exchange cannot occur until the air sac–capillary interfaces are sufficiently thin to permit oxygen diffusion. Such gas exchange was described as 'almost never possible before 23 weeks of gestation but not uncommon after 26 weeks'. Perceptions of the potential for survival are confused by difficulties incurred by imprecisely known gestational age. For example, the survival of infants with very low birthweight may attract media attention without journalistic emphasis that the growth-restricted child was chronologically more mature than suggested by birthweight alone. However, analysis of neonatal survival indicates that survival at 23 weeks' gestation is rare (5–10%), possible at 24–25 weeks (25–35%) and likely only after 26 weeks (> 60%). Unfortunately, the majority of survivors at 23–26 weeks' gestation have significant morbidity (**Q3**).

The management of preterm rupture of membranes is contentious. The use of corticosteriods cannot be strongly supported. Meta-analysis of nine randomized studies suggests that there is a reduction in neonatal respiratory distress syndrome consequent on corticosteroid administration, but no significant reduction in perinatal mortality. There was no significant increase in neonatal infection, although there have been reports of increased maternal endometritis as a result of steroid therapy. The combination of corticosteroid therapy and induction of labour has not been found to be beneficial; no reduction in respiratory distress syndrome occurs, and there is increased neonatal infection (see Crowley). With regard to the use of β-mimetic tocolytic agents in preterm rupture of membranes, the evidence is not encouraging. Meta-analysis does not reveal any benefit of such therapy, and it should probably be restricted to the facilitation of *in utero* transfer to regional centres when necessary. Antibiotic administration in cases of preterm rupture of membranes results in a reduction in deliveries within 1 week, reduced maternal infection before and after delivery, and reduced neonatal infection and pneumonia. However, no reduction in perinatal mortality was found; the results of the ongoing ORACLE study may determine whether a reduction in perinatal mortality can be obtained by antibiotic therapy. Hospitalization has not been demonstrated to be of benefit (**Q4: all false**).

The most important complications of expectant management result from chorioamnionitis. Regular measurement of maternal pulse and temperature, and of fetal heart rate, are mandatory, in order to detect signs of overt infection such as maternal tachycardia, pyrexia, uterine tenderness, purulent vaginal discharge and fetal tachycardia. Covert chorioamnionitis may be detected using serial C-reactive protein estimations and white cell differential counts (although steroid administration produces raised counts), in association with weekly vaginal microbiological cultures. The benefits of amniocentesis to facilitate detection of amnionitis have not been proven. Changes in cardiotocograph tracings and biophysical profile scores appear to correlate with early intrauterine infection. However, at 25 weeks' gestation, these investigations would be extremely difficult to interpret (**Q5**).

The majority of neonatal risks in preterm rupture of membranes relate to prematurity, as in over 80% of cases delivery occurs within 1 week. Although the reported incidence of chorioamnionitis is about 30%, the incidence of neonatal sepsis is much lower (less than 5%). The chance of infection is greatest the earlier the gestational age, and the shorter the latent period before delivery (**Q6: true = B, D; false = A, C, E**).

There is an increasing trend to perform Caesarean section to deliver infants between 24 and 28 weeks' gestation, and this is particularly so when there is a breech presentation. However, evidence to support this trend is lacking. Retrospective and uncontrolled comparisons of vaginally delivered infants and infants delivered by Caesarean section are often subject to selection bias. Nevertheless, the majority of these studies either find no effect of mode of delivery, or suggest that other obstetric variables (principally gestation and birthweight) are of much greater importance. There have been no prospective randomized trials that were sufficiently large and well constructed to produce valid results. When the fetus weighs over 1500 g, there appears to be no advantage in a policy of routine Caesarean section. If such a policy is adopted for infants thought to be below this birthweight with a breech presentation, there will be a number of unnecessary Caesarean sections (congenital abnormalities, inaccurate weight estimation, mistakᶜn presentation), and Caesarean sections will be performed in cases where premature labour was not actually established (**Q7**).

The indications for a classical Caesarean section are few; they include a poorly formed lower segment (as in this case), a non-correctable back-down transverse lie, and some cases of placenta praevia (**Q8**). Unlike the low vertical incision (which might have been preferable in this case), the incision does not involve bladder dissection, and extends from just above the bladder to the uterine fundus. The incidences of both infection and adhesion formation are increased relative to lower segment Caesarean section, as is the risk of uterine rupture in subsequent labours. Moreover, if scar rupture does occur, haemorrhage is greater in the upper uterine segment than in the lower, and the fetus is more likely to be completely expelled from the uterus. Subsequent trials of vaginal delivery are thus contraindicated (**Q9: true = A, B, C; false = D**).

Any woman delivering after preterm rupture of membranes is at increased risk of endometritis, postpartum haemorrhage and venous thrombosis. You should be aware of these risks and consider prophylactic antibiotic and anticoagulant therapy (**Q10**).

REFERENCES

Lockwood CJ. The diagnosis of preterm labor and the prediction of preterm delivery. *Clinic Obstet Gynecol* 1995; **38**: 675–678.

Crowley P. *Cochrane Pregnancy and Childbirth Database (CCPC).* London: BMJ Publishing Group. A regularly updated electronic journal derived from the database of reviews maintained by the Cochrane Collaboration.

FACTS YOU SHOULD HAVE LEARNT . . .

▶ **The diagnosis of preterm rupture of membranes**
▶ **The management of preterm rupture of membranes**
▶ **The indications for, and the implications of, a classical Caesarean section**

SECTION 2

▶ Problems in labour and post delivery

CASE 22

Delay in the first stage of labour

A 25-year-old P1 + 0 Caucasian woman attended the hospital antenatal booking clinic at 18 weeks' gestation. Two years previously she had undergone an elective Caesarean section for placenta praevia at 38 weeks' gestation. This pregnancy had been uncomplicated, and investigations were unremarkable; these investigations included a detailed ultrasound scan which determined that fetal size was consistent with 18 weeks' gestation and the placental site was fundal. She was keen to know how her baby should be delivered as she desired a vaginal delivery.

> **Q1:** When considering the appropriate mode of delivery, which of the following should you plan to do?
> A: Arrange urgent X-ray pelvimetry studies, and review in 2 weeks.
> B: Perform a pelvic examination, determine the pelvic size clinically and make a decision accordingly.
> C: Defer any decision until 37 weeks' gestation.
> D: Provisionally plan for a trial of vaginal delivery without performing any pelvic assessment.
> E: Arrange an elective Caesarean section.

The pregnancy continued to be uneventful, and the patient reattended at a 41 weeks' gestation hospital antenatal clinic visit. The symphysis–fundal height was 39 cm and the presenting part was cephalic with the head engaged.

> **Q2:** Concerning the routine induction of labour at or after 41 completed weeks, which of the following statements are correct?
> A: Recalculation of the estimated date of delivery after early ultrasound scanning significantly reduces the incidence of 'post-term' pregnancies.
> B: Induction of labour reduces the perinatal mortality rate.
> C: Induction of labour increases the maternal use of analgesia in labour.
> D: Induction of labour increases the Caesarean section rate.

> **Q3:** Would you recommend induction of labour in this case and, if so, at what gestation?

The patient was admitted in spontaneous labour on the evening of her antenatal clinic visit. On examination the presenting part was cephalic (two-fifths palpable) and the cervix was 4 cm dilated with intact membranes.

> **Q4:** Would you advocate an amniotomy and, if so, why?

Four hours later, the vaginal examination was repeated, and the cervix was found to be 5 cm dilated. An amniotomy was performed and clear liquor drained. A further 4 hours later, the cervix was reassessed and (as illustrated in Figure 2) found to be 6 cm dilated. Uterine contractions were reported to occur once every 4 minutes. The labour was otherwise uncomplicated, with the liquor remaining clear and the fetal heart rate reactive.

Q5: What abnormal labour pattern is illustrated on the partogram?

Q6: When you review this patient:
  i) What parameters would you assess on clinical examination?
  ii) How would you assess uterine activity?

Q7: Would you recommend augmentation of labour with Syntocinon and, if so, why?

Q8: What Syntocinon regimen would you advocate?

Two hours after a Syntocinon infusion was commenced, a vaginal examination revealed the cervix to be 9 cm dilated. Full dilatation was achieved after a further hour, and, after a short second stage, a female infant weighing 3.67 kg was delivered normally. The postnatal course was uncomplicated.

COMMENTARY

The Cochrane Pregnancy and Childbirth database details that prospective studies of antenatal and intrapartum pelvimetry assessments (either clinical or radiographic) have not been shown to improve outcome. The relatively low risk of malignancy consequent upon fetal exposure to X-rays is avoided by the use of magnetic resonance imaging, but the use of this

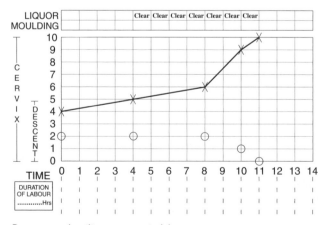

Figure 2   Partogram detailing progress in labour.

technique has not been shown to be helpful. The use of radiological pelvimetry assessment increases the proportion of patients who undergo elective Caesarean section, without decreasing the emergency Caesarean section rate in those deemed suitable for a trial of vaginal delivery. The old adage of 'once a Caesarean, always a Caesarean' has rightly been discredited; even when the previous Caesarean section was adjudged to be due to 'disproportion', many patients achieve a vaginal delivery if allowed to labour. In this case the previous indication for Caesarean section (placental praevia) did not complicate this pregnancy. Thus, as in the majority of patients who have previously delivered by Caesarean section, a well-conducted trial of labour is the optimal management. The woman requested to know how you planned to deliver her baby, and it is good practice to detail a provisional plan at the medical booking appointment. This plan can subsequently be revised, for example if a breech presentation is found at the 37 weeks' hospital or community antenatal clinic visit (**Q1: true = D; false = A, B, C, E**).

In the second trimester, if the gestational age is estimated within 7 days (>2 standard deviations) of that calculated by measurement of the biparietal diameter, then concurrence should be assumed. If the values differ, a repeat ultrasound scan should be performed and, if the ultrasound dates concur, the estimated date of delivery should be recalculated. Using this technique, the incidence of pregnancies reaching 42 completed weeks has been found to be reduced from 11% to 6% (Warsof *et al*, 1983). The Cochrane Centre database includes a meta-analysis of all prospective trials assessing the effects of routine induction of labour at or beyond 41 weeks. These data indicate that induction of labour at this gestation is not hazardous and may reduce the perinatal mortality rate. This benefit seems to be achieved without any increase in intervention (**Q2: true = A, B; false = C, D**). There have been no prospective studies of the effect of induction of labour in 'post-term' pregnancies complicated by a previous Caesarean section. Concerns about augmentation with oxytocics in these patients have led some obstetricians to argue that a decision to perform elective Caesarean section in this group of women (who account for only 1% of antenatal patients) would only minimally increase the overall Caesarean section rate. Others base any decision on patient wishes and the state of the cervix. In this case, the woman was keen to avoid an elective Caesarean section, and a date for induction of labour at 42 completed weeks was arranged (**Q3**).

Over the past 30 years, the practice of early amniotomy has become widespread, as part of a movement associated with the National Maternity Hospital in Dublin. Routine amniotomy is part of a package of care ('the active management of labour') which proponents claim lowers the Caesarean section and instrumental delivery rate, is safer for the baby and is popular with the mother. However, a Cochrane Centre database meta-analysis of six prospective trials found that routine amniotomy had no effect on the Caesarean section and instrumental delivery rate or on measures of fetal or maternal outcome. The only positive effect was a small decrease in the duration of labour. Public suspicions about unnecessary intervention have often threatened to bring the medical profession into disrepute (Sir Anthony Carlisle first voiced these concerns in the British Parliament in 1834), and it is difficult to justify a policy of routine amniotomy (**Q4**).

The partogram (see Figure 2) illustrates primary dysfunctional labour, the commonest pattern of abnormal labour (**Q5**).

A careful abdominal and vaginal examination should be performed. If the fetal head is engaged, well applied to the cervix, and there is no caput or moulding (as was found in this case), then a diagnosis of cephalopelvic disproportion is most unlikely (**Q6i**). Uterine activity can be measured by external or internal tocography. Although the frequency and regularity of uterine contractions can be measured with either method, active contraction area measurements obtained with an intrauterine catheter correlate better with the rate of cervical dilatation than any other parameter (Steer, 1977). However, prospective comparisons of the two methods have failed to show any advantages resulting from the use of intrauterine catheters (reviewed by Arulkumaran and Chua (1994)), and in a busy clinical unit it may be easier, less invasive and cheaper to assess uterine contractions by means of external tocography. There are theoretical advantages to the use of intrauterine pressure monitoring in patients with a previous Caesarean scar; if normal pressure recordings are present, it would seem imprudent to commence oxytocin. Intrauterine pressure measurement has also been recommended in patients with a previous Caesarean scar who are augmented with oxytocin as a sudden decline in uterine activity may be the first and only sign of scar dehiscence (Arulkumaran and Chua, 1994). (**Q6ii**).

Opinion regarding augmentation if there is poor progress in cases of previous Caesarean section varies widely. There are no prospective studies which show an overall increase in scar rupture, yet some obstetricians refuse to augment with oxytocin for fear that scar rupture will occur. On purely logical grounds, in cases such as this, where there is no evidence of disproportion, it would seem reasonable to augment contractions at least to the average level for spontaneous labour. In practice, augmentation may lead to higher levels of uterine activity than normal spontaneous labour (Arulkumaran and Chua, 1994). In addition, a substantial proportion of those who fail to make adequate progress in the first 4 hours of augmentation need operative delivery and are more susceptible to scar rupture. The period of augmentation should probably be limited to 4 hours unless adequate cervical dilatation rates resume (**Q7**).

Published protocols variously recommend a starting dose of 2–6 mU per minute of Syntocinon, with geometric increases every 15–30 minutes. These recommendations were based on *in vitro* studies from which the half-life of Syntocinon was thought to be 3–4 minutes. *In vivo* studies suggest that Syntocinon has a half-life of 10–15 minutes, and obeys first-order kinetics, such that steady plasma concentrations are reached 40–60 minutes after alteration of the infusion. Shorter incremental intervals result in the dose being increased before maximal plasma levels are attained. An incremental interval of 30 minutes is a reasonable compromise between overdosage and the dangers of hyperstimulation on the one hand, and undue delay on the other. Retrospective studies also indicate that a 30-minute incremental interval is optimal, and this interval is consistent with the advice of the American College of Obstetricians and Gynecologists (**Q8**).

REFERENCES

Arulkumaran S, Chua S. Augmentation in labour. In: Ratnam SS, Ng SC, Sen DK, Arulkumaran S (eds) *Contributions to Obstetrics and Gynaecology*, Vol. 3, pp 275–294. London: Churchill Livingstone, 1994.

Steer PI. The measurement and control of uterine contractions. In: Beard RW, Campbell S (eds) *The Current State of Fetal Heart Monitoring and Ultrasound in Obstetrics*, pp 48–70. London: Royal College of Obstetricians and Gynaecologists, 1977.

Warsof SL, Pearce JM, Campbell S. The present place of ultrasound screening. *Clin Obst Gynecol* 1983; **10**: 445–458.

FACTS YOU SHOULD HAVE LEARNT . . .

▶ **The rationale for the induction of labour near 'post-term'**
▶ **The arguments regarding routine amniotomy**
▶ **The arguments regarding the use of (i) intrauterine pressure measurement and (ii) augmentation of labour in cases of previous Caesarean section**
▶ **A rational protocol for the augmentation of labour**

CASE 23

Delay in the second stage of labour

A 27-year-old para 0 + 1 Caucasian woman was admitted to the labour ward in spontaneous labour at 39 weeks' gestation. Her pregnancy had been uncomplicated. She reported good fetal movements and a 30-minute fetal heart tracing was reactive with a rate of 140 beats per minute (bpm). On abdominal examination the symphysis–fundal height was 39 cm, the lie was longitudinal, and the presenting part was cephalic, with two-fifths of the fetal head palpable. On vaginal examination the cervix was 5 cm dilated. An amniotomy was performed and clear liquor drained.

Q1: Would you advocate continuous fetal heart rate monitoring of the baby? If so, why?

Q2: Which of the following statements relating to the use of electronic fetal monitoring (in conjunction with fetal blood sampling) compared with intermittent auscultation are correct?
A: There is an increase in the Caesarean section rate.
B: There is a reduction in the number of infants born with low Apgar scores.
C: There is a reduction in the rate of neonatal seizures.
D: There is a reduction in the rate of admissions to the special care baby unit.
E: There is a reduced incidence of cerebral palsy.

The patient requested an epidural and this was sited. Four hours after admission the vaginal examination was repeated and the cervix was found to be 8 cm dilated. When she was re-examined a further 2 hours later, the fetal head was one-fifth palpable abdominally and, on vaginal examination, the cervix was fully dilated with the fetal head in the left occipitotransverse position. Throughout labour, the liquor remained clear and no fetal heart rate abnormalities were recorded. Active pushing was commenced.

Q3: Do you consider it was appropriate to commence pushing at this time?

After just over 1 hour of active pushing, maternal effort was diminishing and the patient was requesting assistance in delivering her baby. On examination the fetal head was not palpable abdominally. On vaginal examination the fetal position remained left occipitotransverse and there was minimal caput and moulding. The fetal heart rate tracing remained normal and reactive.

Q4: What are the options available for delivering this baby?

The decision was taken to deliver the baby by Kielland's forceps rotational delivery.

Q5: In determining whether this was an appropriate decision, which of the following statements are correct?

A: Rotational forceps deliveries are associated with increased maternal morbidity compared with Caesarean sections.

B: The intelligence quotient (IQ) is lower in children delivered by rotational forceps delivery than in those delivered by Caesarean section.

C: Rotational forceps are associated with a higher failure rate than vacuum extractors.

D: Rotational forceps deliveries are associated with a lower incidence of cephalhaematoma than vacuum deliveries.

Q6: Which of the following are appropriate indications for rotational forceps delivery?

A: The fetal head arrested in the high transverse position.

B: The mentoposterior position with a face presentation.

C: The occipitoposterior position.

D: The fetal head arrested in the deep transverse position.

E: The brow presentation.

Q7: Which of the following are characteristics of Kielland's forceps?

A: A minimal pelvic curve.

B: A sliding lock.

C: A traction handle that is locked over the shanks.

D: A minimal cephalic curve.

Q8: What other rotational forceps are you familiar with?

Q9: Which of the following are prerequisites for a mid-forceps delivery?

A: Fetal head less than one-fifth palpable, regardless of station.

B: Exact position of the fetal head should be known.

C: Complete cervical dilatation.

D: No excessive moulding.

E: An experienced obstetrician to supervise or conduct the delivery.

Q10: What guidelines for mid-forceps delivery would you teach a trainee?

A Kielland's rotational forceps delivery was performed. The fetal head was rotated to the direct occipitoanterior position with ease, and was delivered with two contractions. A female infant weighing 3.41 kg was delivered in good condition. Umbilical cord venous blood samples revealed a pH of 7.29 and a base excess of −6.2. The third stage was uncomplicated, as was the postnatal course.

QII: How would your management have differed in the presence of late fetal heart rate decelerations in the second stage?

COMMENTARY

There is little evidence that continuous fetal heart rate monitoring results in a better outcome than intermittent auscultation. However, in intermittent auscultation, the fetal heart rate should be counted over at least 15 seconds (preferably over 1 minute), and at least every 30 minutes (preferably every 15 minutes). Auscultation should be performed just after a contraction, to detect a persistent deceleration. The frequency of auscultation should probably be increased in the second stage of labour, to take place with each contraction. These guidelines are time consuming and demanding for the birth attendants, particularly if the mother is mobile (**Q1**).

Meta-analysis of randomized trials indicates that the use of electronic fetal monitoring (in conjunction with fetal blood sampling) is associated with a significantly higher Caesarean section rate (increased by about 30%). Most of this increase is in Caesarean sections for 'fetal distress'. There is no benefit of intensive monitoring on neonatal outcome as judged by low or very low Apgar scores, admissions to the special care baby unit, and the perinatal death rate. The one neonatal outcome that does seem to be improved is a reduction in the incidence of neonatal seizures, the importance of which is controversial. This meta-analysis is detailed on the Cochrane Pregnancy and Childbirth Database (CCPC) (BMJ Publishing Group), a regularly updated electronic journal derived from the database of reviews maintained by the Cochrane Collaboration (**Q2: true = A, C; false = B, D, E**).

There have been few randomized controlled comparisons of early versus late pushing in the second stage of labour. These studies provide no evidence to support the limitation of the second stage (i.e. commencing pushing at full dilatation). The only outcome parameter that has been found to be significantly altered is a reduction in the incidence of Kielland's (in some publications the spelling Kjelland is used) forceps rotational deliveries in the group in which pushing was postponed until the vertex was visible at the introitus. There were no differences in the incidence of fetal distress or the degree of perineal trauma (**Q3**).

The options for delivery include Caesarean section, mid-forceps rotational delivery, ventouse or vacuum extraction, and manual rotation followed by non-rotational forceps delivery (**Q4**). There have been no prospective controlled studies of mid-forceps delivery compared with Caesarean section. Any analysis must thus be based on retrospective studies, which are often poorly controlled and poorly interpreted. However, it is difficult to avoid the impression that, compared with delivery by Caesarean section, mid-forceps deliveries may well be associated with short-term benefits regarding maternal mortality, at the expense of increased short-term neonatal complications (Baker, 1995). There is little evidence of longer term neonatal outcome differences resulting from mid-forceps delivery compared with Caesarean section. There is also insufficient evidence to determine whether a mid-forceps delivery is preferable to a mid-vacuum delivery. Unfortunately most of the comparisons between deliveries using forceps and those with vacuum extractors have grouped all forceps together. Meta-analysis of randomized controlled trials indicate that the use of forceps is significantly less likely to fail, more likely to be associated with perineal or vaginal trauma, and less likely to be associated with cephalhaematoma (**Q5: true = D; false = A, B, C**).

Kielland originally recommended the application of his forceps to a head arrested in the high transverse position by a special manoeuvre which involved the anterior blade being passed in front of the fetal head with the concavity of its cephalic curve facing the pubes (Myerscough, 1982). This manoeuvre has been discarded; several cases of rupture of the lower uterine segment followed its use. The high forceps operation has been replaced by Caesarean section. In a mentoposterior position with a face presentation, the chin rarely rotates forward with rotational forceps, and Caesarean section is the best option in the overwhelming majority of cases. Similarly, Caesarean section is the appropriate treatment in a brow presentation. The fetal head arrested in the deep transverse position and the occipitoposterior position are valid indications for the use of rotational forceps (**Q6: true = C, D; false = A, B, E**).

In Kielland's forceps, the pelvic curve is almost eliminated, thus enabling the cephalic grip to be achieved even when the fetal head is in the occipitolateral position. The lock is of a sliding variety which enables the blades to be adjusted if the head is asynclitic (**Q7: true = A, B; false = C, D**). Barton rotational forceps have been advocated in the USA. These forceps (used only when the fetal position is occipitolateral) incorporate a flailed joint in the anterior blade, to enable introduction of the blade between the parietal region of the fetal head and the pubis. The posterior blade has an exaggerated cephalic curve to facilitate introduction into the sacral hollow without damaging the cervix. Other rotational forceps include the Moolgaoker forceps. These differ from Kielland's forceps in that the lock incorporates a distance-spacing wedge. The blades thus maintain a parallel position regardless of the size of the fetal head (Myerscough, 1982) (**Q8**).

All the listed prerequisites are true. In addition, there should be adequate maternal analgesia or anaesthesia, no evidence to suggest either macrosomia or a contracted pelvis, Caesarean section capability and, finally, informed patient consent. The need for a senior obstetrician cannot be overly stressed. The capability to perform a Caesarean section is also imperative. If there is doubt regarding the mode of delivery, the procedure should be performed as a trial in the operating theatre with everything ready for a Caesarean section (**Q9: all true**).

The place of mid-forceps deliveries is undergoing extensive review and critique by obstetricians, the legal profession and the consumer public. If mid-forceps deliveries are performed, then rigorous guidelines should be followed. All the prerequisites detailed above should be fulfilled. If the forceps blades cannot be applied easily, or if the head cannot be rotated with little effort, the procedure should be discontinued and a Caesarean section performed. Only moderate traction throughout a maximum of three contractions should be used. The procedure, antecedents and outcome should be documented. The position, station and condition of mother and baby should be noted. In particular, damage to the maternal genital tract should be described. The practice of sending cord blood samples for pH and blood gas analysis is to be commended (**Q10**).

One particular area of controversy concerns the choice of Caesarean section or mid-forceps delivery in the presence of fetal distress. Despite little evidence to support their contentions, prominent obstetricians have argued for the former in standard texts. However, a Caesarean section in the second stage with an engaged head may result in greater delay and is often a difficult procedure, with considerable maternal and fetal morbidity. Indeed, there have been reports of lower Apgar score after delivery by Caesarean section, compared with mid-forceps delivery, when the indication was fetal distress. Nevertheless, there is some evidence that rotation of the fetal head with forceps produces a deterioration in the fetal acid–base balance (Baker, 1995). This supports the use of fetal blood sampling in the presence of late fetal heart rate decelerations; if the pH is below 7.20, a Caesarean section may well be indicated.

REFERENCES

Baker PN. The place of midforceps deliveries in modern obstetric practice. *Curr Obstet Gynaecol* 1995; **5**: 225–229.

Myerscough PR. The obstetric forceps and the ventouse. In: *Munro Kerr's Operative Obstetrics*, pp 276–294. London: Baillière Tindall, 1982.

FACTS YOU SHOULD HAVE LEARNT . . .

- The evidence for the use of continuous fetal heart rate monitoring
- The indications for rotational forceps delivery
- The characteristics of Kielland's forceps
- Guidelines for the use of rotational forceps

CASE 24

Shoulder dystocia

A 17-year-old P0 + 0 Caucasian woman was admitted to the labour ward in spontaneous labour at 41 weeks' gestation. Her weight at the 18-week booking clinic visit was 67.2 kg and her pregnancy had been uncomplicated. On admission in labour, the symphysis–fundal height was noted to be 44 cm, the lie was longitudinal, the presenting part was cephalic (with three-fifths of the head palpable) and a 30-minute fetal heart tracing was reactive with a rate of 130 beats per minute (bpm). On vaginal examination the cervix was 4 cm dilated. An amniotomy was performed and clear liquor drained.

Four hours later, the vaginal examination was repeated and the cervix was found to be 5 cm dilated with the fetal head in the occipitoposterior position. An intravenous infusion of Syntocinon was commenced. The patient requested an epidural and this was sited. When she was re-examined 4 hours later, two-fifths of the fetal head was palpable abdominally, and on vaginal examination the cervix was 8 cm dilated with the fetal head in the left occipitotransverse position. Three hours later, the cervix was fully dilated with the fetal position unchanged and above the level of the ischial spines. Throughout her labour, the liquor remained clear and no fetal heart rate abnormalities were recorded. Active pushing was commenced.

After 90 minutes of active pushing, there was little progress and the patient was requesting assistance in delivering her baby. On abdominal examination the fetal head was one-fifth palpable. On vaginal examination the position was left occipitoanterior and there was minimal caput and moulding. The fetal heart rate tracing remained normal and reactive. As the fetal head was palpable abdominally, it was decided that any attempted forceps delivery should be in theatre with an anaesthetist and paediatrician present. The epidural was 'topped up' and the patient was transferred to theatre. She was placed in the lithotomy position, catheterized and re-examined; the findings were unchanged. Neville Barnes forceps were applied to the fetal head, and the head was delivered with two contractions, after a right mediolateral episiotomy had been performed. However, the head was then pulled back tightly against the perineum. External rotation of the head did not take place, and gentle downward traction of the head, with moderate fundal pressure, did not accomplish delivery.

QI: What is the incidence of shoulder dystocia?

Q2:   Which of the following pre-pregnancy risk factors suggest an increased likelihood of shoulder dystocia?
A: A history of shoulder dystocia in a previous pregnancy.
B: Diabetes insipidus.

C: Obesity.
D: High maternal birthweight.
E: Nulliparity.

Q3: In this case, would you have predicted shoulder dystocia?

Fortunately, two senior obstetricians, an anaesthetist and a paediatrician were already present. The McRoberts' manoeuvre was performed, i.e. with the help of two assistants, the patient's hips were sharply flexed with her thighs touching the sides of her abdomen. The episiotomy was extended, and suprapubic pressure was applied.

Q4: What are the benefits of:
A: The McRoberts' manoeuvre?
B: Extending the episiotomy?
C: Suprapubic pressure?

Q5: Would you have discontinued fundal pressure?

After 10 minutes, the fetus remained undelivered.

Q6: What would you have done next?

Further attempts to deliver the baby, including an attempt to rotate the posterior shoulder, were unsuccessful, and the obstetricians were faced with three options: symphysiotomy, deliberate clavicular fracture and cephalic replacement (the Zavanelli manoeuvre).

Q7: Which option would you have chosen?

The decision was taken to perform a symphysiotomy. Two assistants again supported the patient's legs to prevent the angle between the legs being greater than 80°. A silver catheter was placed inside the urethra. The catheter (and thereby the urethra) was pushed aside, so that the operator's fingers were in the midline under the symphysis pubis. Using a scalpel, an incision up through the joint was made, commencing at the lower end of the symphysis. Before complete division of the joint, separation of the joint was felt. With suprapubic pressure, and gentle downward traction of the head, delivery of the baby was achieved.

Q8: Do you have any criticisms of the symphysiotomy technique as described above?

A male infant weighing 4.31 kg was delivered. The cord pH was 7.05 and the base excess was -11.1 mEq l^{-1}. The baby cried shortly after delivery and the Apgar score after 5 minutes was 9. The placenta and membranes were delivered intact. After the episiotomy and the extensive vaginal lacerations were sutured, an indwelling catheter was inserted for 5 days. A course of ampicillin and metronidazole was prescribed. The patient made a largely uncomplicated recovery following delivery. Initially she was nursed on her side and, once the catheter had been removed, she commenced mobilization relatively easily. On review 6 weeks after delivery, she was walking without discomfort. Remarkably, her baby suffered no significant complication of the traumatic delivery, with the exception of marked bruising.

Q9: Which of the following statements concerning fetal consequences of shoulder dystocia are correct?

A: The most common palsy seen is Klumpke's palsy, which results in a claw hand.

B: Erb's palsy is due to injury of roots C7, C8 and T1.

C: Resolution of nerve palsies normally occurs within 6–8 weeks.

D: Many fractured clavicles remain clinically undetected.

E: Shoulder dystocia is responsible for 5–10% of term infants who suffer seizures within the first 72 hours of life.

COMMENTARY

The reported incidence of shoulder dystocia varies between 0.2% and 1%, depending on the definition used. Most authors suggest that shoulder dystocia occurs when babies are not delivered after standard measures such as fundal pressure and downward traction on the fetal head, and the anterior shoulder is impacted over the symphysis pubis. Severe shoulder dystocia occurs when both shoulders remain over the pelvic inlet (**Q1**).

Fetal weight increases with advancing parity, thus nulliparity is not a risk factor. If labour is permitted in a pregnancy following a history of shoulder dystocia, the recurrence risk is about 10%. A previous history of a macrosomic infant is an important risk factor, and may be associated with maternal obesity or abnormal glucose intolerance. Infants of mothers with diabetes mellitus are more than twice as likely to suffer shoulder dystocia as similar birthweight infants of non-diabetic mothers. The relationship between maternal and infant birthweight is significant; maternal birthweight is an independent predictor of infant macrosomia (**Q2: true = A, C, D; false = B, E**).

There were certain features of this labour that are typical of shoulder dystocia. The patient was admitted after her estimated date of delivery, and on examination the symphysis–fundal height was increased. Although clinical estimation of fetal weight is an inexact science, the symphysis–fundal height measurement suggested an infant of above-average birthweight. The risk of shoulder dystocia in infants weighing less than 4 kg is 0.07%, whereas in infants over 4 kg the risk rises to 1.3%. This risk increases to 23% in infants weighing over 4 kg after a prolonged second stage and mid-pelvic delivery (Benedetti and Gabbe, 1978). However, most cases of shoulder dystocia occur in infants of average weight and one in five cases have no predictive factor. In most cases, shoulder dystocia is an unexpected finding which could not have been foreseen. Many parents find it difficult to accept that the degree of trauma associated with shoulder dystocia could not have been predicted, and medicolegal claims are commonplace. Successful litigation by the plaintiff is uncommon, the basic rule being that the defendant's liability is confined to reasonably foreseeable dangers and that 'the occurrence of shoulder dystocia was not an injury of a class or character foreseeable as a possible result of . . . failure by the obstetrician' (James, 1991) (**Q3**).

The advantage of the McRoberts' manoeuvre is that rotation of the symphysis pubis occurs in an upward direction. This reduces the angle of inclination of the pelvic brim and encourages the anterior shoulder to slip from behind the symphysis pubis. Extension of the episiotomy should reduce the pressure around the fetal neck, lower fetal cerebral engorgement and aid any manual manoeuvres. The aim of suprapubic pressure is to rotate the shoulders transversely so that they are in alignment with the transverse (and widest) diameter of the inlet. It is important to recognize that the mechanism of shoulder dystocia is one of failure of shoulder rotation into the transverse position with a consequent inability to accommodate to the shape of the pelvis (**Q4**). Unless the anterior shoulder has been displaced, fundal pressure will be ineffective and may be harmful, resulting in increased neurological or bony injuries to the fetus (**Q5**).

All staff working on the labour ward must be familiar with a clear protocol for shoulder dystocia. The next manoeuvre attempted was Wood's screw manoeuvre, the aim of which is to dislodge the anterior shoulder manually. In the presence of suprapubic pressure, the operator's hands attempt to rotate the posterior shoulder towards the fetal chest, thus dislodging the anterior shoulder from above the symphysis. Following the failure of this manoeuvre, an attempt was made to deliver the posterior shoulder by passing a hand into the sacral hollow. The plan was to flex the fetal elbow and forearm, sweep the fetal arm across the chest and deliver the arm. The delivered arm is then used as a tractor to pull the posterior arm forwards and allow the anterior shoulder to enter the pelvis. However, there was insufficient space for the operator to pass a hand into the sacral hollow to reach the elbow (**Q6**).

A combination of McRoberts' manoeuvre, suprapubic pressure, Wood's screw manoeuvre and attempts to deliver the posterior shoulder should result in the delivery of most cases satisfactorily. Failure of the above techniques means that the degree of shoulder dystocia is severe, and that the outcome for the baby is poor. Three 'desperate' procedures are described: symphysiotomy, clavicular fracture and cephalic replacement (the Zavanelli manoeuvre). Each of these options has serious disadvantages. Symphysiotomy is not a procedure familiar to most UK obstetricians. Deliberate clavicular fracture or cleidotomy is not known to be effective and is potentially dangerous because of the underlying subclavian vessels. Uterine rupture is a potential complication of the Zavanelli manoeuvre, in which the head is replaced under anaesthesia and delivery is effected by Caesarean section (**Q7**).

Neither of the obstetricians present had seen a symphysiotomy procedure before this case, and their technique differed from that described by more experienced operators (Van Roosmalen, 1991). It is, indeed, important to prevent abduction of the legs during and after symphysiotomy, in order to prevent straining of the sacroiliac joints. Likewise, the urethra should be moved away from the midline. However, a solid-bladed scalpel should be used, otherwise fragments of the blade can be left in the fibrocartilage of the joint. The preferred technique is an incision at the junction of the upper and middle thirds of the joint, traversing the joint with the blade until the point is felt impinging on the vagina by the underlying finger of the left hand. The upper third should then be used as a fulcrum against which the scalpel is levered to incise the lower two-thirds. The remaining third of the symphysis should then be cut after reversing the scalpel by 180° (Van Roosmalen, 1991) (**Q8**).

Shoulder dystocia can result in either generalized asphyxia or local trauma (neurological damage or fractures). Neurological damage results from a combination of fundal pressure and downward traction on the head injuring the cervical nerve roots. Erb's palsy (C5–7) is most commonly seen, although Klumpke's palsy can result from extension to C7, C8 and T1. Horner's syndrome (due to coincidental damage to the sympathetic chain), and phrenic nerve palsy (C3–4) are less common sequelae. Resolution of nerve palsies normally occurs within 6–8 weeks. The most common fracture is a fracture of the clavicle – many fractured clavicles remain clinically undetected and are detected only when a tender swelling over the affected clavicle is noted (**Q9: true = C, D, E; false = A, B**).

REFERENCES

Benedetti TJ, Gabbe SG. Shoulder dystocia: a combination of fetal macrosomia and prolonged second stage of labour with midpelvic delivery. *Obstet Gynecol* 1978; **52**: 526–531.

James CE. Medico legal problems: shoulder dystocia. *Curr Obstet Gynaecol* 1991; **1**: 117–118.

Van Roosmalen J. Symphysiotomy – a reappraisal for the developing world. In: Studd J. (ed.) *Progress in Obstetrics and Gynaecology*, Vol. 9, pp 149–162. Edinburgh: Churchill Livingstone, 1991.

FACTS YOU SHOULD HAVE LEARNT . . .

▶ **The risk factors for shoulder dystocia**
▶ **A clear management strategy for coping with shoulder dystocia**
▶ **The preferred technique of symphysiotomy**
▶ **The fetal consequences of shoulder dystocia**

CASE 25

Emergency Caesarean section

A 19-year-old P0+0 Asian woman was admitted to the labour ward at 39 weeks' gestation, complaining of regular uterine contractions and after having noted that her membranes had ruptured. Her pregnancy had been uncomplicated. The fetal heart rate was regular, at approximately 140 beats per minute (bpm), and meconium staining of the amniotic fluid was noted. The symphysis–fundal height was 39 cm, the lie was longitudinal and a cephalic presenting part was noted with the fetal head one-fifth palpable. On vaginal examination the cervix was 4 cm dilated and a vertex presentation confirmed the position was occiputoposterior. Four hours later, the findings on vaginal examination were unchanged, and a Syntocinon infusion was commenced. No fetal heart rate abnormalities were noted.

> **Q1:** **Which of the following parameters of a fetal heart rate in the first stage of labour are consistent with a normal cardiotograph?**
> A: A baseline of 160 bpm.
> B: A baseline variability of 20 bpm.
> C: 4 accelerations in 20 minutes.
> D: The absence of accelerations for 20 minutes.
> E: A baseline of 110 bpm.

> **Q2:** **Which of the following statements concerning Syntocinon augmentation of labour are correct:**
> A: Unless hyperstimulation occurs, fetal PO_2 is unaffected by uterine activity.
> B: Oxytocin infusion rates greater than 12 mU per min are associated with uterine hyperstimulation in 30–40% of cases.
> C: Unless hyperstimulation occurs, the inter-contraction interval has little effect on fetal oxygenation.
> D: Oxytocin infusions should not be commenced if there is any fetal heart rate abnormality.
> E: Oxytocin infusions should be discontinued if there is any fetal heart rate abnormality.

Shortly after the Syntocinon infusion commenced, persistent variable fetal heart rate decelerations were noted. A fetal blood sample was taken and the pH was found to be 7.26 with a base excess of -6.2 mEq l^{-1}.

> **Q3:** **Which of the following statements concerning the use of fetal blood sampling in labour are correct?**
> A: It is associated with a reduction in Caesarean sections for fetal distress.
> B: It is associated with improved neonatal outcome.

C: It is necessary in the presence of meconium.

D: It may be helpful in pregnancies complicated by Rhesus disease.

E: It may be helpful in pregnancies complicated by diabetes.

Ten minutes after fetal blood sampling, a rise in the fetal heart rate to 170 bpm was noted, followed by a sudden persistent bradycardia at 60 bpm. After a vaginal examination to exclude umbilical cord prolapse, the decision to perform an urgent or 'stat' Caesarean section was taken.

Q4: How quickly should a 'stat' or urgent Caesarean section be performed?

Q5: What actions should medical/midwifery staff take whilst awaiting the theatre team?

Q6: Which of the following statements concerning anaesthesia for emergency Caesarean sections are correct?
A: General anaesthetic inhalation agents isoflurane and enflurane promote uterine relaxation and thus increase bleeding.
B: Failed intubations occur in approximately 1 in 300 cases.
C: Spinal anaesthesia is associated with decreased maternal morbidity.
D: Regional anaesthesia is associated with increased postoperative backache.
E: Bupivacaine is toxic at lower plasma concentrations than lignocaine.

The patient was taken to the operating theatre, where, under a general anaesthetic, a lower segment Caesarean section was performed. A viable 2.90 kg female infant was delivered with Apgar scores of 2 and 9 at 1 and 5 minutes respectively. Meconium was successfully aspirated and the baby responded well to intermittent positive pressure ventilation. No cause for the bradycardia was found. The pH of an umbilical artery sample was 7.14, with a base excess of -10.2 mEq l^{-1}. The interval from the decision to perform a Caesarean section to delivery of the baby was 13 minutes. However, the routine administration of prophylactic antibiotics was inadvertently omitted.

The patient made a good postoperative recovery until 36 hours after delivery, when she was noted to have a temperature of 38.9°C, with an associated tachycardia. General examination was unremarkable, although uterine tenderness was noted. A diagnosis of endomyometritis was made.

Q7: What criteria should you use to diagnose endomyometritis following Caesarean section?

Q8: Which of the following statements concerning post-emergency Caesarean section endomyometritis are correct?
A: In the absence of prophylactic antibiotics, the incidence is over 30%.
B: The incidence is fivefold to tenfold higher than after a vaginal delivery.
C: Prophylactic antibiotics reduce the incidence by 30%.
D: In about 10% of cases, concurrent bacteraemia will occur.

Q9: **Which of the following are typical pathogens in post-Caesarean section endomyometritis?**

A: *Escherichia coli.*

B: *Proteus mirabilis.*

C: *Gardnerella vaginalis.*

D: *Staphylococcus aureus.*

E: *Klebsiella pneumoniae.*

Q10: What antibiotic regimen would you instigate?

The patient was commenced on antibiotic therapy. Blood and urine cultures were negative. Within 48 hours of antibiotics, she was apyrexial and clinically well. She was discharged home on the sixth postoperative day and the postoperative recovery was otherwise uncomplicated.

COMMENTARY

Characteristics of a normal or reassuring cardiotocograph (CTG) in the first stage of labour include: two or more accelerations (more than 15 bpm for more than 15 seconds) in 20 minutes, a baseline fetal heart rate between 110 and 150 bpm, and a baseline variability between 5 and 25 bpm. The absence of accelerations for more than 40 minutes would be characteristic of a 'non-reactive' CTG and worthy of suspicion (**Q1: true = B, C, D, E; false = A**).

Every uterine contraction above 6 kPa produces a cessation in maternal intervillous placental blood flow, and thus produces relative hypoxia for the fetus. Fetal Po_2 falls by 0.5–0.75 kPa with each contraction; the lowest Po_2 being at the end of the contraction. Recovery of the fetal Po_2 takes 60–90 seconds – this is the time taken to replace the oxygen-depleted maternal pool of blood. The total period of reduced oxygenation (contraction plus recovery time) is up to 2.5 minutes. This emphasizes the importance of adequate inter-contraction intervals, and oxytocin infusions can result in iatrogenic fetal hypoxia. The data sheet supplied with Syntocinon states that it should not be administered in the presence of fetal distress. If any fetal heart rate abnormality occurs during an infusion, the infusion should be discontinued (**Q2: true = B, D, E; false = A, C**).

Meta-analysis of randomized trials indicates that the use of fetal blood sampling in labour is associated with a reduction in Caesarean sections for fetal distress. There is no clear benefit of the use of fetal blood sampling as assessed by Apgar score, neonatal seizures, admission to the special care baby unit or the incidence of cerebral palsy. If the fetal heart rate is normal, neonatal outcome is similar in the presence or absence of meconium; thus fetal blood sampling is not necessary. However, if the fetal heart rate pattern is abnormal, the presence of meconium in labour is associated with a higher chance of the baby being acidotic, born in poor condition and needing resuscitation at birth. Fetal blood sampling may be used to monitor blood glucose levels in pregnancies complicated by diabetes, and haemoglobin, blood group and Coombs' test in pregnancies complicated by rhesus disease (**Q3: true = A, D, E; false = B, C**).

The appropriate time interval from the decision to perform a Caesarean section to delivery will vary with the clinical situation. The American College of Obstetricians and Gynecologists (1985) has recommended a maximum time interval of 30 minutes. However, more expeditious response may often be necessary. In the fetal monkey a complete occlusion of the umbilical cord will result in a drop of pH by 0.04 per minute and of base excess by $1 \text{ mEq l}^{-1} \text{min}^{-1}$. Thus, in a previously unasphyxiated term fetus, up to 8 minutes of total hypoxia may not cause permanent brain damage; longer periods with partial asphyxia can result in a good outcome. Examples in obstetric practice which can be compared with the totally asphyxiated fetal monkey include cord prolapse, uterine rupture, vasa praevia and massive placental abruptions. In these conditions, delivery within 8 minutes is desirable; there are few centres that can consistently achieve deliveries within this time. Situations in which delivery within 15–30 minutes is acceptable include persistent fetal heart rate decelerations and abnormal presentations late in the first stage of labour (**Q4**).

Unless already *in-situ*, an intravenous cannula should be inserted and blood should be taken (for a full blood count and either grouping and saving of serum or cross-matching). Informed written consent should be obtained. The patient should be given an antacid (for example, 30–60 ml sodium citrate) to reduce the morbidity associated with aspiration pneumonitis, regardless of the anaesthetic employed. The Syntocinon infusion should be discontinued. Transport to the operating suite should be initiated as soon as possible, particularly if the labour ward is not contiguous with the theatre suite. A urethral catheter can be inserted and the abdomen shaved. Preoxygenation with 100% oxygen utilizing a clear anaesthetic mask, tilting the patient to facilitate lateral displacement of the uterus, will expedite induction of anaesthesia if a general anaesthetic is to be used. In cases where fetal distress is present with hyperstimulation or regular uterine activity, and when a rapid decision to delivery interval cannot be achieved, tocolysis with a β-agonist may be helpful (**Q5**).

Unless an epidural has already been sited, the options for anaesthesia for an emergency Caesarean section are either general or spinal anaesthesia. General anaesthesia, utilizing rapid sequence induction and endotracheal intubation, retains a role in obstetrics. In most cases a short-acting barbiturate coupled with succinylcholine is used to accomplish intubation. Cricothyroid pressure is maintained until the airway is secure in order to minimize the risk of aspiration during induction. A mixture of nitrous oxide and oxygen is then used until the umbilical cord is clamped. Then it is customary to add a low-concentration inhalation agent (isoflurane or enflurane) which does not promote uterine relaxation or increased bleeding. Emergency Caesarean sections may require general anaesthesia when severe antepartum haemorrhage has occurred or if a coagulopathy is known or suspected. Severe fetal bradycardia is a relative indication for general anaesthesia, but is a rare event occurring in less than

10% of emergency Caesarean sections. Spinal anaesthesia has become the method of choice for emergency Caesarean sections as a result of the maternal, fetal and neonatal disadvantages that are inherent in the technique of general anaesthesia. Maternal disadvantages include the risk of failed intubation (reported to occur in 1 in 300 cases), which may be followed by the aspiration of stomach contents, and the lack of maternal awareness of the birth. Maternal postoperative morbidity is decreased by spinal anaesthesia, in particular, blood loss is reduced by almost 50%. The fetal and neonatal advantages result from improved placental perfusion, greater sympathoadrenal activity in the neonate and less central nervous system depression. Long-term backache is increased twofold after regional analgesia in labour, but this is likely to be due to poor posture, as there is no increased incidence after Caesarean section under regional compared with general anaesthesia. The main toxic reactions to spinal anaesthetic drugs involve the central nervous and cardiovascular systems. These reactions usually follow accidental intravenous injection, or use of excessive doses. Signs and symptoms of central nervous system toxicity include lightheadedness, numbness of the tongue, visual disturbances, unconsciousness and convulsions. Bupivacaine is toxic at lower doses than lignocaine, and there have been case reports of cardiac arrest following bupivacaine administration (**Q6: true = B, C, E; false = A, D**).

Any patient who is found to have pyrexia and uterine tenderness after Caesarean section should be presumed to have endomyometritis until proven otherwise, especially if there are suggestive results such as a raised white blood count. Pyrexia is generally defined as a temperature of 38°C on two occasions, after the first 24 postoperative hours. This 24-hour period was advocated to prevent overdiagnosis as a result of dehydration, pulmonary atelectasis, etc. In practice, these conditions rarely cause pyrexia after a Caesarean section, and any temperature of 38°C should probably be considered significant. You should be able to distinguish between uterine tenderness and the normal surgical tenderness of an abdominal incision. Manual pressure above the umbilicus should enable you to palpate the uterine fundus without encroaching on the lower abdominal incision (**Q7**).

While the incidence of puerperal endomyometritis is considerably less than 5% in women delivering vaginally, it is between 35 and 40% after Caesarean section if prophylactic antibiotics have not been given. Meta-analysis of the use of prophylactic antibiotics indicates that this therapy results in a major and significant reduction in the incidence of febrile morbidity due to endomyometritis, wound infections and other serious infections after Caesarean section (see Smaill). The incidence of postoperative endomyometritis is reduced by over 50%. In approximately 10% of cases, concurrent bacteraemia will accompany post-Caesarean endomyometritis. Risk factors for the development of postoperative endomyometritis include young maternal age, a long labour, prolonged ruptured membranes and multiple vaginal examinations (**Q8: true = A, B, D; false = C**).

The bacteria involved in the pathogenesis of post-Caesarean endomyometritis are usually derived from inhabitants of the patient's cervicovaginal flora. Most studies describe a mixture of aerobic bacteria (such as *Escherichia coli, Klebsiella pneumoniae, Proteus mirabilis*, group B streptococcus and the enterococcus), anaerobic Gram-positive cocci (such as peptococcus and peptostreptococcus) and anaerobic Gram-negative bacilli (such as *Bacteroides* and *Gardnerella vaginalis*). Therefore antibiotics that are active against both aerobes and anaerobes are appropriate (**Q9: true = A, B, C, E; false = D**).

The 'gold standard' of antibiotic therapy for post-Caesarean endomyometritis is the combination of clindamycin and an aminoglycoside (usually gentamicin). The clindamycin provides anaerobic and some aerobic Gram-positive coverage, whilst gentamicin is active against most commonly encountered Gram-negative aerobes. Alternatives include substitution of metronidazole or chloramphenicol for clindamycin, substitution of aztreonam for gentamicin, a combination of penicillin plus gentamicin and metronidazole, or one of the extended-spectrum penicillins such as ampicillin–salbactam. If a cephalosporin had been given as prophylaxis, a penicillin should have been used owing to the possibility of enterococcus infection (**Q10**).

REFERENCES

American College of Obstetricians and Gynecologists, Committee on Obstetrics. Maternal and fetal medicine. *ACOG Newsletter* February 1985.

Smaill F. *Cochrane Pregnancy and Childbirth Database (CCPC).* **(London: BMJ Publishing Group). A regularly updated electronic journal derived from the database of reviews maintained by the Cochrane Collaboration.**

FACTS YOU SHOULD HAVE LEARNT . . .

▶ The characteristics of a normal cardiotocograph in the first stage of labour
▶ The value of fetal blood sampling in labour
▶ The advantages of the different options for anaesthesia for an emergency Caesarean section
▶ How to diagnose and manage post-Caesarean endomyometritis

CASE 26

Caesarean hysterectomy

A 32-year-old married P2+0 Pakistani woman booked in the hospital antenatal clinic at 14 weeks' gestation. She had had an uncomplicated full-term normal delivery and an elective Caesarean section for placenta praevia at 38 weeks' gestation. The Caesarean section had been uncomplicated and she had not required a blood transfusion. At 18 weeks' gestation an ultrasound scan revealed a low-lying placenta. Her blood group was O Rh positive, with no red cell antibodies, and her full blood count was normal with a haemoglobin concentration of 11.1 g dl^{-1}. There was no evidence of haemoglobinopathy or thalassaemia. She had not experienced any vaginal bleeding.

Q1: How would you counsel her and what advice would you offer her general practitioner and midwife?

Q2: Which of the following statements regarding the Confidential Enquiry into Maternal Mortality 1991–93 are correct?
A: Maternal deaths from haemorrhage increase with maternal age.
B: The maternal death rate from haemorrhage was 6.4 per 100 000 maternities and fell with respect to the previous report.
C: There were 150 direct deaths attributable to haemorrhage.
D: Consultant obstetricians are recommended to be present in the cases of placenta praevia and previous Caesarean section.
E: Common mistakes in management which classified the care as substandard included under-estimation of blood loss, delay in blood transfusion, and delay in consultant involvement.
F: The commonest causes of death were (in order): thromboembolism, hypertension, haemorrhage, early pregnancy problems.

A further ultrasound scan was organized at 34 weeks' gestation. The patient was advised to return immediately if there was any vaginal haemorrhage. The pregnancy proceeded without complication and at the repeat ultrasound scan a grade IV placenta praevia was noted. The fetus was appropriately grown.

The patient was admitted to hospital and counselled about the proposed delivery and the possibility for the need of a Caesarean hysterectomy. At no time during the pregnancy had she experienced any vaginal bleeding. An elective Caesarean section was performed at 39 weeks' gestation.

Q3: What preparations and planning should you make for the operation?

Following delivery of the baby, the placenta was noted to be adherent in the lower segment of the uterus. Attempts to deliver the placenta resulted in dramatic haemorrhage which could not be stopped. A hysterectomy was performed with an estimated blood loss of 5 litres, and 8 units of cross-matched blood were transfused.

Q4: What surgical difficulties and complications may be encountered during and after this type of operation?

In the early postoperative period the blood pressure remained stable at 100/60 mmHg and the pulse rate was 100 beats per minute (bpm). Pulse oximetry revealed an oxygen saturation of 97% on 4 litres per minute of nasal oxygen therapy.

Q5: Why is it important to maintain the haemoglobin oxygen saturation above 95%?

The patient remained stable and was transfused with a further 3 units of blood. Her urine output remained satisfactory with no haematuria. The vaginal loss was heavy but did not increase in amount and there were no signs of microvascular bleeding (i.e. bleeding from mucous membranes, generalized petechiae, oozing from wound or venepuncture sites).

Q6: What investigations would you arrange at this point?

Q7: Which of the following statements about stored blood are correct?

A: Modern anticoagulant preservatives ensure adequate red cell concentrations of 2,3-diphosphoglycerate and therefore ensure oxygen-carrying capacity for up to 14 days after blood collection.

B: There are practically no functioning platelets after 48 hours' storage.

C: Factor VIII levels decrease in stored blood to 50% after 24 hours and down to 30% at 5 days.

D: Factor V activity falls to 50% in 14 days.

E: Various red cell preparations may themselves precipitate disseminated intravascular coagulation.

The results of investigations revealed prolonged bleeding times, including an activated partial thromboplastin time (APTT) of 120 (control 30) s, prothrombin time of 42 (control 13) s and thrombin time of 45 (control 10) s. The platelet count was $35 \times 10^9 \ l^{-1}$ and the haemoglobin concentration was $9.0 \ g\,dl^{-1}$.

Q8: What is the diagnosis and what should be done to correct this problem?

Q9: Which of the following statements regarding the coagulation mechanism are correct?

A: The thrombin time measures the rate of conversion of fibrinogen to fibrin.

B: A Factor V Leiden gene defect produces a defect in the intrinsic arm of
the clotting cascade which is measured by the prothrombin time.
C: Cholestasis of pregnancy can produce a prolonged prothrombin time.
D: Heparin in therapeutic doses produces prolongation of the extrinsic
arm of the clotting cascade (measured by the APTT).
E: Placenta praevia and pre-eclampsia are causes of coagulopathy in
pregnancy.

Fortunately the coagulopathy was corrected with the replacement
therapy and no further bleeding was encountered. The baby was breastfed
and she made a complete recovery. At the postnatal visit the vaginal vault
was well healed. The histology of the uterus revealed placenta increta.

COMMENTARY

In cases of a low-lying placenta at 18 weeks' gestation, patients should be
informed that the 'after-birth' is over the womb's outlet and that, if any
vaginal bleeding is experienced, they should seek medical advice
immediately. You should also provide reassurance that most of the low-
lying placentae become fundal later in pregnancy. A re-scan will be
necessary in the third trimester. The woman's general practitioner and
midwife should be notified and asked to re-refer her back to the hospital if
any vaginal haemorrhage is experienced (**Q1**).

The Confidential Enquiry into Maternal Mortality 1991–1993 (1996) is a
very important document and you should incorporate the data from the
enquiry in any examination answer. In addition, the information and
recommendations should influence your everyday clinical practice.
Maternal deaths from haemorrhage do increase with maternal age and did
fall with respect to the previous report. The maternal death rate from
haemorrhage for 1991–1993 was 6.4 per 1 000 000 maternities. There were
15 direct deaths attributable to haemorrhage, and consultant obstetricians
are recommended to be present in the cases of placenta praevia and
previous Caesarean section. The common mistakes in management which
classified the care as substandard did include under-estimation in blood
loss, delay in blood transfusion, and delay in consultant involvement. The
commonest causes of death were (in order): thromboembolism (15.5% of
cases), hypertension (14%), early pregnancy problems (14%), haemorrhage
(11.6%) (**Q2: true = A, D, E; false = B, C, F**).

Before the operation the anaesthetist should be informed of the
potential risks and a general, rather than a regional, anaesthetic should be
employed in the event of maternal hypotension. Six units of blood should
be cross-matched and available in theatre at the start of the operation and
the preoperative haemoglobin concentration should be more than
11.0 g dl^{-1}. A consultant obstetrician should perform the procedure or
should at least be readily available, and the operation planned at a
convenient time for laboratory and other staff in the event of complication
(**Q3**).

The main surgical difficulties of a Caesarean hysterectomy concern identification of the cervix and ensuring good haemostatic technique especially when dealing with the vaginal vault. Pedicles should be double tied and the peritoneum closed with adequate drainage of the pouch of Douglas. The ureters should be identified from the pelvic brim through their pelvic course to the bladder. Internal iliac artery ligation should be considered if pelvic haemorrhage persists. The complications that may be encountered during the operation include damage to visceral structures, haemorrhage and haematoma formation. Postoperative complications include sepsis, thrombosis, paralytic ileus and bowel obstruction. Nasogastric suction should be employed with slow return to normal intake once bowel sounds are audible (30 ml of fluid per hour until flatus is passed). Opiates should be limited as much as possible. Pneumatic boots and compression stockings are of proven benefit in reducing postoperative thrombosis. Chest physiotherapy and early mobilization are essential to prevent atelectasis and infection. Stress ulceration of the stomach and haemorrhage should be considered, and prophylaxis with an H_2-receptor inhibitor like ranitidine or cimetidine. Psychological support is important and the possibility of postnatal depression should be considered (**Q4**).

The relationship between the oxygen saturation and partial pressure is a sigmoid curve with a critical point at which small decreases in the partial pressure result in a large fall in haemoglobin oxygen saturation. This is known as the oxygen dissociation curve. The critical point is around a saturation of 85–90% and so, to avoid denaturation of haemoglobin, you must endeavour to keep the partial pressure at a level such that the oxygen saturation is over 95% (**Q5**).

The minimum laboratory investigations required in this patient are: haemoglobin concentration or packed cell volume (PCV), platelet count, clotting studies (thrombin time, prothrombin time, APTT); and baseline urea, electrolytes, calcium and albumin levels. You should aim to keep the haemoglobin level above 10 $g\,dl^{-1}$ (or the PCV above 0.2 l/l) and the platelet count above $50 \times 10^9\,l^{-1}$ (**Q6**).

All the statements about stored blood are true (Hewitt and Machin, 1990), and they highlight the fact that with massive blood transfusion all you are providing is blood volume and red cell oxygen-carrying capacity. Platelets and clotting factors have to be considered and added to prevent further blood loss (**Q7: true = A, B, C, D, E**).

The patient had developed a coagulopathy, probably a consumptive coagulopathy, but there may have been an element of disseminated intravascular coagulation. The blood transfusion and coagulation laboratories must be notified and a specialist haematologist should be involved in the management. Fibrinogen levels should be measured and replacement of clotting factors and platelets given with the following guidelines: fresh frozen plasma – 4 units (1 litre) as bolus, cryoprecipitate – 10 units as a bolus (2–2.5 g fibrinogen should be given when the plasma fibrinogen level is below 1 $g\,l^{-1}$, which should increase the plasma fibrinogen level by $1g\,l^{-1}$); platelets – 5–10 units as bolus or 1 unit of concentrate per 10 kg bodyweight (each unit has a minimum of 55×10^9 platelets). In this case the fibrinogen level was 0.78 g l^{-1} and was corrected with replacement therapy (**Q8**).

The thrombin time does measure the rate of conversion of fibrinogen to fibrin. Factor V Leiden gene defect does not produce a defect in the intrinsic arm of the clotting cascade but prevents the binding of activated protein C, a natural anticoagulant, to Factor V. Cholestasis of pregnancy can produce a prolonged prothrombin time (which tests the intrinsic arm of the coagulation cascade), which may be corrected with vitamin K. Heparin in therapeutic doses does cause prolongation of the extrinsic arm of the clotting cascade, and its action is monitored by measurement of the APTT. Abruption and pre-eclampsia are causes of coagulopathy in pregnancy (**Q9: true = A, C, D; false = B, E**).

REFERENCES

Hewitt PE, Machin SJ. ABC of Transfusion. Massive blood transfusion. *BMJ* 1990; **300**: 107–109.

Report on Confidential Enquiries into Maternal Deaths in the United Kingdom 1991–1993. London: HMSO, 1996.

FACTS YOU SHOULD HAVE LEARNT . . .

▶ **The recommendations of the Confidential Enquiry into Maternal Mortality regarding haemorrhage**
▶ **The complications of Caesarean hysterectomy**
▶ **The management of massive haemorrhage**

CASE 27

Obstetric shock

A 29-year-old P3 + 0 Caucasian woman had a normal delivery of a 3.5 kg infant with an estimated blood loss of 200 ml at the time of delivery. When she was discharged home the following day, she was breastfeeding and was asymptomatic. The puerperium was uncomplicated until day 10 when she began to feel unwell with some lower abdominal pain and a slight increase in the lochia. The following day the vaginal bleeding became heavier and she called the community midwife. Having assessed the patient, the midwife consulted the duty obstetric registrar at the local hospital. The midwife conveyed the history and stated that the woman had probably lost in excess of 1 litre of blood, she looked pale, her pulse rate was 92 beats per minute (bpm) and her blood pressure was 100/60 mmHg.

Q1: **What would your advice be to the attendant midwife?**
A: Call the general practitioner to visit.
B: Send the woman directly to the local hospital for assessment.
C: Arrange an urgent outpatient appointment to see the consultant.
D: Commence oral antibiotics and re-assess in 6 hours.
E: Put the patient to bed and re-assess in the morning.

Q2: **What is the diagnosis and what do you think are the possible causes of the problem?**

The paramedical ambulance was summoned; an 18-G intravenous cannula was inserted in the forearm and an infusion of normal saline was commenced. On arrival at the hospital you are called to see the patient.

Q3: **What are the important features of the history and examination that you need in order to assess the seriousness of the case?**

On examination, the woman was pale and her pulse rate was 88 bpm but thready in character, her blood pressure was 100/60 mmHg, her abdomen was soft, and she had a moderate vaginal loss. The uterus was involuted and tender and the cervix was closed. Shortly after arrival, she collapsed with a pulse rate of 104 bpm and a blood pressure of 60/0 mmHg.

Q4: **Which of the following should be included in your plan for the treatment or investigation of this patient?**
A: To arrange theatre space for an urgent evacuation of the uterus.
B: To arrange an ultrasound scan and administer intravenous ergometrine 500 µg.

C: To resuscitate the patient with colloids and oxygen by mask.
D: To organize a full blood count and a cross-match of whole blood.
E: To pack the vagina and catheterize the urinary bladder.

Once the woman was resuscitated, reassessment revealed a pale woman with a blood pressure of 120/70 mmHg and a pulse rate of 92 bpm, cold extremities and only a moderate vaginal blood loss. Oxygen saturation by pulse oximetry was Sao_2 of 90%, with 25% oxygen by facial mask. A full blood count revealed a haemoglobin concentration of 11.3 $g\,dl^{-1}$, a platelet count of $444 \times 10^9\,l^{-1}$, and a white cell count of $15.5 \times 10^9\,l^{-1}$.

Q5:   What are the most likely diagnoses at this stage and what investigations would you perform?

Q6:   What are the most likely microorganisms to be responsible for secondary postpartum haemorrhage?
A: *Chlamydia trachomatis*
B: *Escherichia coli*
C: *Bacteroides*
D: Streptococci
E: *Actinomyces*
F: *Neisseria gonorrhea*

Q7:   What antibiotics would you administer?

Augmentin 1.2 g was administered intravenously. Within 30 seconds of administration of the antibiotic, the woman started to experience breathing difficulties. She became restless and developed an urticarial skin rash. Her pulse rate was 120 bpm and her blood pressure was 70/45 mmHg. Pulse oximetry revealed that the haemoglobin oxygen saturation was 60%.

Q8:   What do you think the most likely diagnosis is now?
A: Septicaemic shock
B: Waterhouse–Friderichsen syndrome.
C: Anaphylactic shock.
D: Venticular tachycardia following acute myocardial infarction.
E: Pulmonary embolism.

Q9:   Which of the following would your management now include?
A: Calling a senior anaesthetist urgently.
B: Administration of dexamethasone 12 mg intravenously.
C: Administration of a further dose of antibiotics.
D: Administration of parenteral adrenaline.
E: Arranging an electrocardiogram (ECG) and inserting a central venous pressure (CVP) line.

Q10: **What antibiotics will you institute to deal with the intrauterine infection that caused the original problem?**

The contemporaneous blood transfusion was suspended. At this stage the haemoglobin concentration was 8.9 g dl^{-1}, the platelet count was $180 \times 10^9 \text{ l}^{-1}$ and her coagulation profile was normal.

Q11: **What are you going to do about the blood transfusion?**
A: Cancel the transfusion and give oral iron treatment.
B: Return the blood to the laboratory, inform the laboratory of the problem and continue the transfusion later.
C: Re-cross-match 4 units of blood.
D: Recommence the transfusion once the patient is stabilized.
E: Check the hepatitis status of the patient.

The patient subsequently had an uncomplicated recovery with bed rest, multiple antibiotic therapy and blood transfusion. She left hospital 2 days later with a haemoglobin concentration of 11.6 g dl^{-1}. No organisms were isolated and no further haemorrhage occurred.

Q12: **What are you obliged to tell the patient and the patient's general practitioner? Are there any other institutions that should be informed or consulted?**

COMMENTARY

The midwife's observations of a blood loss in excess of 1 litre demand that the woman is brought to hospital immediately. In general, a young fit woman can compensate and maintain her blood pressure for a long time before it drops. It is often appropriate to double estimations of blood loss, and a pulse rate of 92 bpm may indicate a compromised patient. The woman must be assessed by an experienced obstetrician who is in a position to treat any blood loss but, more importantly, be able to treat any *further* blood loss (**Q1: true = B; false = A, C, D, E**).

The diagnosis is one of secondary postpartum haemorrhage. The two most common causes are of retained products of conception and intrauterine infection. Primary postpartum haemorrhage is blood loss of 500 ml or more after the birth of the baby for the first 24 hours; secondary haemorrhage is classified from this point until 6 weeks. This condition is common and probably accounts for a large proportion of the 500 000 maternal deaths that occur worldwide each year (**Q2**).

Assessment of a patient with a secondary postpartum haemorrhage requires a review of the hospital notes and delivery records, and of the baby. It is an important point and a reminder that you should always check the baby's notes as vertical infection may give an indication of any causative organism for intrauterine infection. Questioning first-hand observers (relatives and the midwife) about the amount of loss is important. Never underestimate the value of taking the pulse yourself (for at least 30 seconds); remember: history, examination and investigation. In this case the woman had decompensated suddenly and these processes have to be carried out quickly. It is important to realize that a young fit woman can compensate remarkably well even with a normal pulse rate. Lying and sitting or standing blood pressure readings may provide a clue to compensated hypovolaemia and is a valuable observation (**Q3**).

This woman required urgent resuscitation with colloids and oxygen by mask, and she needed a blood transfusion. A general anaesthetic would probably have been fatal at this stage, and intravenous ergometrine would also have been da⁻.gerous. An ultrasound scan would have been inappropriate and time wasting as the diagnosis in this scenario was a clinical one. A vaginal pack was contraindicated as it would only have hindered further assessment of blood loss; however, a urinary catheter would have been sensible to monitor urine output and renal function (**Q4: true = C, D; false = A, B, E**).

As the uterus was involuted and tender, and the cervix was closed, the diagnosis must be intrauterine infection rather than retained products of conception. You should have taken endocervical swabs for culture and sent blood cultures. You must exclude the complications of puerperal sepsis, which include acute renal failure and coagulopathy including thrombocytopenia. The putative anaemia should be treated with blood transfusion, with 2 units always available in the event of a recurrent vaginal haemorrhage (**Q5**).

The most likely microorganisms to invade the uterus, placental bed and spiral arteries are those that inhabit the vagina, i.e. anaerobes including *Bacteroides* and peptostreptococci, and the enteropharyngeal group (*E. coli* and streptococci, including *Streptococcus faecalis*, β-haemolytic streptococcus and *S. viridans*) (**Q6: true = B, C, D; false = A, E, F**).

Your choice of antibiotics must be broad spectrum to include the enteropharyngeal organisms and, most importantly, to cover for the anaerobes. An ideal choice would be: ampicillin 1 g intravenously 6 hourly and metronidazole 1 g per rectum 8 hourly (rectal administration is much cheaper than intravenous administration and the drug is well absorbed rectally). It is important to check the patient's allergy status. In fact a swab from the baby's eye revealed a *S. viridans* isolate, of which the woman's general practitioner had been informed. Unfortunately, the result had not been filed in the case notes, a potentially serious mishap and a fact that may have helped considerably in the acute situation described in this case. Careful review of the hospital case notes is an important and often rewarding activity (**Q7**).

Anaphylactic reaction is an immunological description of a type 1 hypersensitivity reaction following immunoglobulin (Ig) E or IgG release from mast cells and results in acute histamine secretion with resultant bronchospasm, hypotension and urticarial skin reaction. In Gram-negative septicaemia, the rash is petechial in type. Waterhouse–Friderichsen syndrome is acute haemorrhage into the adrenal gland, usually as a terminal event, and may rarely occur in neonates following hypoxic ischaemic encephalopathy (**Q8: true = C; false = A, B, D, E**).

Acute anaphylaxis is an acute medical emergency and the treatment is 0.5 ml adrenaline 1/1000 intramuscularly, subcutaneously or submucosally followed by hydrocortisone 100 mg intravenously with colloid fluids (Fisher, 1995). It would seem sensible to get some help from an expert in resuscitation, especially as this patient has been in shock on two occasions from two different causes (**Q9: true = B, D; false = A, C, E**).

The question of antibiotics following the anaphylactic reaction to the Augmentin should be discussed with the duty microbiologist, but multidrug therapy will be required. Metronidazole intravenously or rectally is mandatory for the anaerobes and an aminoglycoside (gentamicin, vancomycin, tobramycin, netilmicin) for the enteropaths. Meta-analysis has suggested that single daily dose regimen are as effective as multiple daily dose regimens, with less nephrotoxicity, no greater risk of ototoxicity and greater convenience at a lower cost (Barza et al, 1996). The quinolones (e.g. ciprofloxacin) are more expensive but give good cover for the pharyngeal streptococci, which the penicillins and third-generation cephalosporins would normally cover but which are contraindicated in this case. The allergic cross-reaction with penicillin and cephalosporins is about 10% (**Q10**).

The patient remained anaemic and needed to have a haemoglobin concentration greater than 11 g dl^{-1} in order to have some reserve in the event of further vaginal haemorrhage. The patient's blood was screened for unusual antiplatelet antibodies which may cause transfusion reactions; this proved negative and a 6-unit transfusion continued without complication (**Q11: true = B; false = A, C, D, E**).

The primary care team, in this case the general practitioner, must be informed about the anaphylactic reaction to the drug Augmentin. It would be extremely useful for the patient to know what component of the drug induced the acute allergic reaction, and a referral to an immunologist or specialist in allergy should be seriously considered. In addition, the general practitioner should be asked to check her blood for the development of red cell antibodies following the transfusion, as this may be useful in subsequent pregnancies or for emergencies. The problem of hepatitis C should be considered following a transfusion of more than 4 units of blood. In countries where rigorous screening of donated blood is not employed by transfusion services, human immunodeficiency virus (HIV) must also be considered. In the UK, the Committee on Safety of Medicines should be informed of the adverse drug reaction through the process of the yellow notification forms.

REFERENCES

Barza M, Ioannidis JPA, Cappelleri JC, Lau J. Single or multiple doses of aminoglycosides: a meta-analysis. *BMJ* 1996; **312**: 338–345.

Fisher M. Treatment of acute anaphylaxis. *BMJ* 1995; **311**: 731–733.

FACTS YOU SHOULD HAVE LEARNT . . .

▶ The emergency management of postpartum haemorrhage
▶ The differential diagnosis of secondary postpartum haemorrhage
▶ The treatment of acute anaphylaxis

CASE 28

Puerperal seizures

A 32-year-old para 1 + 2 Caucasian woman had an uncomplicated pregnancy and, after a spontaneous labour at 39 weeks' gestation, delivered a male infant in good condition. Both the patient and her son had an uneventful postpartum course until the 8th day following delivery. Whilst resting at home, she experienced generalized tonic–clonic seizures. Her husband contacted her general practitioner who advised him to call an ambulance and stated that he would attend as soon as possible. The ambulance and the general practitioner arrived simultaneously. The general practitioner found her to be comatose, with a blood pressure of 130/70 mmHg. Her husband confirmed that she had never previously had any seizures and that the pregnancy had not been complicated by pre-eclampsia. An intravenous cannula was inserted, and the general practitioner accompanied her in the ambulance to the hospital.

On admission to hospital, the patient remained comatose and was unresponsive to pain. The blood pressure was 130/75 mmHg and the axillary temperature was 36.8°C. The respiratory rate was 24 per minute, and there was no evidence of peripheral or central cyanosis. On neurological examination, her pupils were equally round, although sluggishly reactive to light. Her eyes were tonically deviated to the right and the corneal response was absent. Motor examination revealed generalized hypotonicity without fasciculations. No myoclonic jerks were seen. Deep tendon reflexes were markedly decreased. No clonus was found. A positive Babinski reflex was noted. On examination of the optic fundi, no papilloedema was seen.

Q1:   What is your emergency management of this comatose patient?

A 1.2g loading dose (20 mg kg^{-1}) of phenytoin (diluted in 100 ml normal saline) was infused intravenously over 45 minutes.

Q2: Would you advocate anticonvulsant therapy?

Q3: What are the advantages of phenytoin as the anticonvulsant choice?

Q4: Which of the following should be included in your differential diagnosis of puerperal seizures?
A: Amniotic fluid embolism.
B: Eclampsia.
C: Pheochromocytoma.
D: Thrombotic thrombocytopenic purpura.
E: Guillain-Barré syndrome.
F: Anthrax.

The haemoglobin level was reported as $13.8\ g\,dl^{-1}$ and the white blood cell count as $36.2 \times 10^9\ l^{-1}$ (predominantly lymphocytes). Plasma levels of glucose and of all electrolytes were within the normal range. Computed tomography (CT) of the head was carried out and a lumbar puncture was performed. The results of both studies were entirely normal.

Q5: How do these results help you to establish a diagnosis?

An electroencephalogram was essentially normal, although occasional lateralized epileptiform discharges in the right posterior temporoparietal region were noted. Visual evoked potentials were normal. Magnetic resonance imaging (MRI) was performed and revealed cortical vein thrombosis and cortical vein infarct in the posterior parietal area.

Q6: What is the incidence of cortical vein thrombosis in pregnancy, and how does it more typically present?

Q7: What is the aetiology of cerebral venous thrombosis?

Q8: When considering management of this patient, which of the following statements are correct?
A: The mortality rate associated with the condition is over 50%.
B: All patients should be anticoagulated.
C: All patients should receive antihypertensive therapy.
D: If the initial event is survived, long-term sequelae are uncommon.

The patient's level of consciousness gradually improved over the next 12 hours, and when she was examined the following day a neurological examination was entirely normal. After 48 hours of intravenous phenytoin therapy, a daily dose of 300 mg was prescribed for 2 months. The patient suffered no further complications, and when reviewed at a 6-week follow-up visit, she was asymptomatic and examination findings were unremarkable.

COMMENTARY

In the emergency management of this comatose patient, the integrity of her airway must first be assured. The relaxed pharyngeal musculature of the postictal state may potentially combine with vomit or blood in the upper airway, leading to airway obstruction, asphyxia and cardiac arrest within minutes. Her mouth and pharynx should be cleared of any foreign matter, and her head extended to prevent hypopharyngeal obstruction by the base of the tongue. Intubation is not usually necessary, because the duration of the postictal state is usually brief. Supplementary oxygen should be given. Any comatose patient should be closely observed to ensure that adequate ventilation is occurring. If the aetiology of the seizures is uncertain, a bolus of glucose should be given. Continuous cardiac monitoring and pulse oximetry should be instigated, and blood pressure should be regularly checked. Venous access should be established, and venous blood drawn for the appropriate laboratory tests (**Q1**).

Repeated seizures of whatever cause can result in brain damage and can create life-threatening systemic disturbances. Maintenance therapy with a long-acting anticonvulsant should start immediately. It will usually take over 30 minutes to administer sufficient long-acting anticonvulsant to be effective, so diazepam should be at hand if seizures recur in the interim (**Q2**). Phenytoin is a credible anticonvulsant of choice, with several advantages. It is safe to use; serious side-effects such as arrhythmias and hypotension are rarely seen in young women if the infusion rate is not excessive; and it does not depress consciousness. It is simple to administer and therapeutic circulating levels are achieved in 30–60 minutes. Its central mechanism is understood, and it is of proven efficacy in epilepsy. One possible disadvantage of phenytoin therapy is that it has not been shown to prevent eclamptic fits (**Q3**).

There are a myriad of potential causes of puerperal seizures. Approximately 30% of eclamptic fits occur after delivery; although there have been reports of eclamptic fits more than 1 week postpartum, they are generally within the first 48 hours after birth. In this case, the absence of hypertension, or of any history of pre-eclampsia, also makes this diagnosis unlikely. Non-obstetrically related causes of seizures include epilepsy, pseudoseizures secondary to hysteria, syncope or hyperventilation. They also include central nervous system disease such as meningitis, intracranial haemorrhage or tumours, cerebral venous thrombosis, ruptured berry aneurysm, hypertensive encephalopathy and skull trauma. Certain medical diseases such as phaeochromocytoma, and metabolic disorders (hyponatraemia, hypoglycaemia), water intoxication, thyroid disease, and thrombotic thrombocytopenic purpura have all been associated with seizure activity. In a patient immediately following delivery, anaesthetic drug toxicity is a particularly important cause (**Q4: true = B, C, D; false = A, E, F**).

Many of the uncommon metabolic disorders are excluded by the normal electrolyte and glucose levels. A raised white cell count would be consistent with meningitis, but there was an absence of meningeal signs and the cerebrospinal fluid assessment was unremarkable. There was no sign of any cerebral tumour, ruptured aneurysm or arteriovenous malformation on the CT scan (and the cerebrospinal fluid was not blood stained). A normal CT scan does not exclude a cerebral venous thrombosis; failure of CT to reveal venous thrombosis is well recognized (**Q5**).

The incidence of cerebral venous thrombosis in pregnancy is approximately 1 in 5000 pregnancies (Amias, 1970), but is much higher in the Indian subcontinent. Most cases occur in the puerperium, and are within 5 weeks of delivery. Thrombotic obstruction of the superior sagittal sinus or cortical veins produces increased intracranial pressure and impaired cerebrospinal fluid absorption. The primary presenting symptom in the majority of cases is thus a severe headache; nausea and vomiting, blurred vision and impaired intellect are also typical symptoms. Acute bilateral papilloedema may develop and pyrexia is characteristic. It is the subsequent regional cerebral infarction that results in focal neurological signs or seizures (**Q6**).

The aetiology of cerebral venous thrombosis is uncertain. Embolization of a pelvic thrombus is one suggested cause, but this seems unlikely on an anatomical basis. Others have suggested that cerebral venous thrombosis is related to Virchow's triad, recognizing that venous stasis, vascular wall damage and a hypercoagulable state are all associated with pregnancy and delivery. In addition, other hypercoagulable states such as malignancy and oral contraceptive use are predisposing factors in cerebral venous thrombosis, as are hyperviscosity syndromes such as sickle cell haemoglobinopathy and dehydration. Some studies suggest that the pathophysiology may be related to arachidonic acid metabolites and their influence on platelet aggregation and endothelial cell behaviour. Associations with hereditary protein C deficiency, antithrombin III deficiency and lupus anticoagulant have also been reported. These thrombotic tendencies are discussed further in case 3 (**Q7**).

Although mortality rates of up to 30–45% have been reported (Amias, 1970), most recent reports suggest that most women recover, and that for those that survive the initial event there are few residual neurological deficits. The principles of management are to manage any case of cerebral venous thrombosis jointly with an obstetrician and either a neurologist or a neurosurgeon, to control seizures and to attain adequate hydration. Anticoagulation had been advocated, but is associated with a risk of death from intracranial haemorrhage, and there is no evidence for a reduction in mortality with anticoagulant therapy (Levine *et al*, 1988). Reduction of intracranial pressure with high-dose steroids will sometimes by indicated. The use of antihypertensive agents is also controversial, because hypertension is thought to be a major compensatory mechanism. A variety of other agents, including aspirin, fibrinolytic agents and dextran, have also been suggested, although most reports are anecdotal (**Q8: true = D; false = A, B, C**).

REFERENCES

Amias AG. Cerebral vascular disease in pregnancy: occlusion. *Journal of Obstetrics and Gynaecology of the British Commonwealth* 1970; **77**: 312–325.

Levine SR, Twyman RE, Gilman S. The role of anticoagulation in cavernous sinus thrombosis. *Neurology* 1988; **38**: 517.

FACTS YOU SHOULD HAVE LEARNT . . .

▶ The emergency management of a comatose patient
▶ The differential diagnosis of puerperal seizures
▶ The typical presentation of cerebral venous thrombosis
▶ How to manage cerebral venous thrombosis

SECTION 3

◗ **Gynaecological problems**

CASE 29

Amenorrhoea

A 43-year-old P1 + 1 married Caucasian woman presented to her general practitioner with 3 months' amenorrhoea, hot flushes and night sweats. She had had a salpingo-oöphorectomy some years before for an ectopic pregnancy and subsequently conceived spontaneously after two years without using contraception. The pregnancy and delivery were uncomplicated. There was no past history of pelvic inflammatory disease or postpartum haemorrhage. General and pelvic examination was normal and her body mass index was 25 kg m^{-2}. The couple were using barrier methods for contraception.

Q1: What is your diagnosis at this stage?
    A: The menopause.
    B: The climacteric.
    C: Secondary amenorrhoea.
    D: Oligomenorrhoea.
    E: Cryptamenorrhoea.

Her general practitioner performed some investigations: a pregnancy test was negative, thyroid function tests were within the normal range, serum oestradiol concentration was less than 20 pmol l^{-1}, follicle stimulating hormone (FSH) level was 69.4 U l^{-1} and prolactin concentration 238 mU l^{-1}.

Q2: What is your diagnosis now?
    A: The menopause.
    B: The climacteric.
    C: Resistant ovary syndrome.
    D: Hypogonadotrophic hypogonadism.
    E: Hypo-oestrogenaemia.

Hormone replacement therapy was commenced (conjugated oestrogens 0.625 mg daily plus norgestrel 150 µg for 12 days each month) and the patient was given advice about contraceptive needs at this stage in her life.

Six months later she complained of heavy periods and was found to have an abdominal mass arising from the pelvis.

Q3: What would you do next?
    A: Liver function tests and a serum CA125 level.
    B: Hysteroscopy and/or dilatation of the cervix and uterine curettage.
    C: Laparotomy for a definitive diagnosis.
    D: Catheterize the urinary bladder and examine.
    E: None of the above.

An ultrasound scan was performed and revealed a twin pregnancy of approximately 14 weeks' gestation. She was asked to stop her hormone replacement therapy and an appointment was made for her to see a consultant obstetrician.

Q4:   Is this pregnancy most likely to be monozygotic or dizygotic?

A subsequent ultrasound scan revealed a single anterior placenta with two male fetuses and a thin amniotic septum dividing the fetuses.

Q5:   How would you counsel the woman regarding prenatal diagnostic tests?

After consultation an uncomplicated chorionic villus sampling was performed and a 46XY karyotype was identified by direct count and culture.

Q6:   What are the risks to this pregnancy and what are the greatest threats to the well-being of the fetuses?

At 23 weeks' gestation she was admitted to hospital with a 2-day history of abdominal pains and a 3-week history of increasing abdominal distension. On examination the abdomen was distended and tense, and the symphyseal–fundal height was 34 cm. On vaginal examination the cervix was closed.

Q7:   What is the probable diagnosis?

Q8:   What treatment options are available?

Amnioreduction was arranged for the following day. However, labour commenced that night. A rapid delivery of a 620 g male baby was followed by an assisted breech delivery of a 359 g male baby with no signs of life. The third stage of labour was completed with the delivery of a single placenta with no postpartum haemorrhage. The first twin died after 24 hours with severe prematurity and necrotizing enterocolitis. At autopsy the placentation was confirmed as monochorionic and diamniotic, and the twins were monozygotic. Twin one had visceromegaly when compared with the other twin who had Potter's facies consistent with oligohydramnios and was growth restricted. A twin–twin transfusion was confirmed.

Six months after the delivery, the patient was still grieving for the loss of her twin boys. She had not had a period, had no galactorrhoea and was experiencing hot flushes and severe night sweats. Findings on examination were normal and her body mass index was 24 kg m^{-2}.

Q9:   What investigations would you perform?

Investigation results included the following: FSH 85.7 U l^{-1}, luteinizing hormone (LH) 50.4 U l^{-1}, prolactin 195 mU l^{-1}, serum total oestradiol 135 pmol l^{-1}.

Q10: What is the diagnosis?
A: Sheehan's syndrome.
B: Kallmann's syndrome.
C: Asherman's syndrome.
D: Ovarian failure.
E: Chiari–Frommel syndrome.

Q11: What treatment would you offer if this menopausal pattern persisted after 3 months?

COMMENTARY

At her initial presentation, the condition should strictly be described as oligomenorrhoea. You are obliged to exclude pregnancy as a cause for the oligomenorrhoea and a previous history of ectopic pregnancy should have heightened your awareness of the fact. With the symptom profile described, it would be reasonable to investigate further to exclude the possibility of ovarian failure, thyroid disease and hyperprolactinaemia rather than waiting. Secondary amenorrhoea is the cessation of menstruation for more than 6 months, although some authorities quote 12 months (**Q1: true = D; false = A, B, C, E**).

When reviewing the investigation results, caution must be applied with single results, especially as the woman was 43 years of age. The menopause is by definition a clinical, not a laboratory, diagnosis: 12 months' amenorrhoea at the end of the reproductive life of a woman. A biochemical diagnosis of menopausal ovarian failure can be confirmed only when the FSH level is greater than 30 U l^{-1} on two occasions at least 3 months apart. The tests could reflect the onset of ovarian failure due to a lack of follicles available for recruitment (the climacteric). Resistant ovary syndrome is confined to women below 35 years of age (**Q2: true = B, E; false = A, C, D**).

The old surgical adage concerning abdominal masses gives a differential diagnosis of: fat, fluid, flatus, faeces, fetus, full bladder and ovarian tumour. Therefore, an ultrasound scan is probably the optimal investigation at this stage to diagnose the nature of the abdominal mass (**Q3: true = E; false = A, B, C, D**).

Multiple pregnancies in women over 40 years old are most commonly the result of a double ovulation and so are dizygotic, all of which are diamniotic and dichorionic. The diagnosis of chorionicity is discussed further in case 19. The ultrasound scan was able to determine only that the pregnancy was diamniotic (**Q4**).

In this case, the premise that the pregnancy is monozygotic makes the issue of fetal karyotyping straightforward: either by chorionic villus sampling from the anterior placenta or by amniocentesis. The former has the advantage of an immediate result from a direct preparation of the placental cells enabling a chromosome count to confirm euploidy of the cells. The cell culture may on occasions (1%) give rise to placental mosaicism, and necessitate subsequent amniocentesis or fetal blood sampling to resolve the fetal karyotype. There is an increase in the risk of miscarriage, which for chorionic villus sampling is quoted at 2–4% and for amniocentesis about 1–2% but may be higher in twin pregnancies, up to 3.6%. For dizygotic twins the issue is far more complicated in obtaining individual fetal tissue. The woman needs to understand the complicated implications of a twin pregnancy with one twin euploidy and the other aneuploidy. As far as this woman was concerned, she wanted to know whether at least one child was of normal karyotype (**Q5**).

All the complications for singleton pregnancies are increased in a twin pregnancy but the greatest risks to the fetus are preterm labour and delivery, and the risk of twin-to-twin transfusion (**Q6**).

The probable diagnosis at the time of admission was a twin–twin transfusion and an ultrasound scan would confirm the diagnosis. In this case the scan revealed a large-for-dates twin with polyhydramnios and a smaller 'stuck' twin (**Q7**).

Dexamethasone (12 mg intramuscularly on two occasions) should be administered because it is the single most effective therapeutic intervention for reducing the risk of respiratory distress in the preterm neonate, and also reduces the risk of intracranial haemorrhage and necrotizing enterocolitis (betamethasone has also been used successfully). Another option which remains unproven in randomized trials is amnioreduction to reduce the intrauterine distension and pressure. This may prevent preterm labour and improve the prognosis for the 'stuck' donor twin with oligohydramnios. Indomethacin has been used medically to reduce polyhydramnios but this drug reduces renal blood flow and alters cerebral flow. Moreover, premature closure of the ductus arteriosus may seriously compromise the smaller 'donor' twin. β-Sympathomimetic tocolytics are dangerous drugs and in the presence of polyhydramnios are probably ineffective. After careful consideration, β-sympathomimetic therapy may be appropriate to allow time for steroids to become effective. Another intervention available, again of unproven value, is laser ablation of the interconnecting placental vasculature (**Q8**).

In this case, after 6 months' amenorrhoea, you should check the gonadotrophin levels (FSH and LH), oestradiol and prolactin levels, and perform thyroid function tests (**Q9**).

Sheehan's syndrome is secondary amenorrhoea after childbirth complicated by massive postpartum haemorrhage. The biochemical evidence would have suggested Sheehan's syndrome if the FSH, LH and oestradiol levels had been low or unrecordable. Chiari–Frommel syndrome is continued lactation with hyperprolactinaemia (greater than 1000 mU l^{-1}); computed tomography or magnetic resonance imaging of the pituitary fossa is required to exclude a prolactinoma or microadenoma. Asherman's syndrome is unlikely without any uterine instrumentation, although severe endometritis following Caesarean section has been known to obliterate the endometrial basal layer. Hysteroscopy would exclude that diagnosis. Kallmann's Syndrome is excluded by the lack of anosmia and is usually a cause of primary amenorrhoea. As the values for FSH and LH were high and the oestradiol level was low, you must consider ovarian failure as the diagnosis (**Q10: true = D; false = A, B, C, E**).

Oestrogen replacement therapy should be considered to treat the patient's menopausal symptoms and to prevent ischaemic heart disease and osteoporosis. The minimum therapy required to protect against osteoporosis is as follows: oral ethinyloestradiol 15 μg per day, oral oestradiol 2 mg per day, oral conjugated oestrogens 0.625 mg per day, transdermal patches 50 mg per patch. This patient requires progestogens for 12 days each month to prevent endometrial hyperplasia and adenocarcinoma (**Q11**).

FACTS YOU SHOULD HAVE LEARNT . . .

▶ **The differential diagnosis of secondary amenorrhoea**
▶ **The investigation of a patient with secondary amenorrhoea**
▶ **The complications of twin pregnancies**
▶ **The management of twin–twin transfusions**

CASE 30

Oligomenorrhoea

A 22-year-old married P0+0 Pakistani woman presented with a three-year history of oligomenorrhoea (three to four periods a year) and a desire to conceive. Her menarche was at the age of 12 years and she reported a regular menstrual pattern until the age of 19 years. She had never used any contraception and had been married for 3 years. Her past medical history was largely unremarkable, although she suffered mild asthma. The couple had not experienced any problems with sexual intercourse and there was no past history of any sexually transmitted diseases. There was no family history of diabetes and the relationship was not consanguineous.

> **Q1:** **Which of the following is the most likely cause for this couple's inability to conceive?**
> A: Precocious puberty.
> B: Fallopian tube disease and blockage.
> C: Azoospermia.
> D: Infrequent ovulation.
> E: Polycystic ovary syndrome.

> **Q2:** **What features of the woman's examination are of particular importance in this case?**

On examining the woman, no abnormalities were found; her body mass index was within the normal range (21 kg m^{-2}). Examination of her husband was also normal.

> **Q3:** **What investigations would you perform at this stage?**

The full blood count showed a haemoglobin level of 11.0 g dl^{-1} with a mean corpuscular volume (MCV) of 62.1 fl (normal range 76–97 fl) and a mean corpuscular haemoglobin (MCH) of 19.4 pg (normal range 27–32 pg). Iron studies and haemoglobin electrophoresis were performed. The haemoglobin electrophoresis showed two bands, haemoglobin A and A$_2$ bands with 6.0% of the haemoglobin content as A$_2$ (normal range 2.3–3.3%). Iron studies did not show any evidence of iron deficiency.

> **Q4:** **What are the genetic implications for this couple?**

Semen analysis was normal. An ultrasound scan of the ovaries showed multiple small follicles, the largest of which was 7 mm. A progesterone challenge test of medroxyprogesterone 10 mg per day for 5 days was positive.

On day 5 of the menstrual cycle the results shown in Table 2 were obtained.

TABLE 2 RESULTS OBTAINED ON DAY 5 OF THE MENSTRUAL CYCLE		
Analyte	Result	Normal range
Luteinizing hormone (LH)	14.6 IU l⁻¹	1–26 IU l⁻¹
Follicle stimulating hormone (FSH)	5.1 IU l⁻¹	1–10 IU l⁻¹
Prolactin	490 mU l⁻¹	< 650 mU l⁻¹
Sex hormone binding globulin (SHBG)	30 nmol l⁻¹	50–80 nmol l⁻¹
Testosterone	1.8 nmol l⁻¹	1.7–2.8 nmol l⁻¹
Androstenedione	8.5 nmol l⁻¹	4–10 nmol l⁻¹
17-Hydroxyprogesterone	17.0 nmol l⁻¹	0.9–3.0 nmol l⁻¹
Dihydroepiandrostenedione sulphate	6.2 μmol l⁻¹	3.3–8.2 μmol l⁻¹
Thyroxine	12 pmol l⁻¹	10–20 pmol l⁻¹
Thyroid stimulating hormone (TSH)	1.3 mU l⁻¹	0.5–5.5 mU l⁻¹

Q5: What are the possible diagnoses and what confirmatory tests would you advocate?

Q6: Which of the following statements about 17-hydroxyprogesterone are correct?
A: It exhibits a nyctohemeral variation.
B: It varies throughout the menstrual cycle.
C: Is raised in 21-hydroxylase-deficient states.
D: Is a precursor hormone of the zona fasciculata of the adrenal gland.
E: Heterzygotes for classical and non-classical congenital adrenal hyperplasia have a mild deficiency which may be diagnosed only by measuring 17-hydroxyprogesterone on adrenocorticotrophic hormone (ACTH) stimulation testing.

The patient did not respond to induction of ovulation with clomiphene citrate up to a dose of 100 mg daily from day 2 to 6 of the menstrual cycle. An uncomplicated laparoscopy revealed a normal pelvis and genital organs with patent fallopian tubes following dye hydrotubation.

Q7: Which of the following statements concerning clomiphene citrate are correct?
A: Clomiphene citrate is an oestrogen receptor modulator which used to be known as an antioestrogen.
B: The multiple pregnancy rate with its use is approximately 30%.
C: It is indicated in women with chronic anovulation for any cause.
D: A common side-effect is headache.
E: The maximum recommended dose is 250 mg per day in the luteal phase of the cycle.

Q8: What form of gonadotrophin preparation would you recommend at this stage to induce ovulation?

Ovulation induction with 75 units of human menopausal gonadotrophin (HMG) daily resulted in multiple folliculogenesis. In view of the risk of multiple pregnancy and ovarian hyperstimulation syndrome, two such cycles were abandoned.

Q9: What are the recommended precautions when using gonadotrophins to induce ovulation and what are the possible side-effects?

Subsequently, the patient was given 250 µg dexamethasone at night until the 17-hydroxyprogesterone was suppressed. She was then prescribed alternate-day doses of pure FSH (75 units). After 1 week, the dose of FSH was increased to daily injections. On day 21 of the cycle there were two follicles of 15-mm diameter, the serum oestradiol level was 1445 pmol l^{-1} and the serum LH level was 6.0 U l^{-1}.

Q10: How would you manage the ovulation from this point?

She did not receive FSH the following day, and the next day there were two follicles of 18-mm diameter. Human chorionic gonadotrophin (hCG) 10 000 units was administered and the couple was encouraged to try to conceive. The patient did not menstruate and at 7 weeks' gestation a singleton intrauterine pregnancy was noted.

Q11: Would you recommend continuing the dexamethasone?

The dexamethasone was continued until 20 weeks' gestation and then the dose was slowly reduced over 2 weeks when it was stopped. The pregnancy was uncomplicated and culminated in the delivery of a live male infant at term.

COMMENTARY

In this case the most obvious cause for the delay in conception is the infrequent ovulation. More information is required to establish the cause of the chronic anovulation (**Q1: true = D; false = A, B, C, E**). A careful examination will often provide you with clues as to the origin of the patient's anovulation. The body mass index (BMI), expressed as a ratio of weight (kg)/height (m^2), is essential as low bodyweight is a common and potent cause of hypothalamic and ovarian dysfunction. In contrast, a raised BMI is associated with polycystic ovaries. An objective score of female hair growth as described by the Ferriman–Gallwey score (1961) may suggest excess androgen production, as may signs such as acne and evidence of seborrhoea. You should always check for thyroid enlargement and for expressed galactorrhoea. Moreover, in cases of infertility, it is essential to examine the male partner (**Q2**).

The essential initial investigations at initial presentation included analysis of the husband's semen, determination of the patient's rubella immune status and a full blood count. An ultrasound scan would be helpful in the assessment of ovarian function and to determine whether the ovaries were polycystic, multicystic or atrophic in appearance. A series of hormonal tests should be performed in cases of chronic anovulation: prolactin (which should not be measured the same day as the examination), thyroid function tests, gonadotrophins FSH and LH. The following sex steroids should also be measured: testosterone, androstenedione, 17-hydroxyprogesterone, dihydroepiandrostenedione sulphate (DHEAS) and sex hormone binding globulin (SHBG). A test of tubal patency will be required at some stage (**Q3**).

β-Thalassaemia is an autosomal recessive condition in which the production of the β chain of haemoglobin is reduced. If her husband carries a trait for any haemoglobinopathy or thalassaemia, any offspring may be seriously affected. He thus needs to have haemoglobin electrophoresis studies. These were performed and a normal electrophoretic pattern was observed. If he had been affected, the couple would have been counselled about these possibilities and the availability of prenatal testing (**Q4**).

The results of the investigations performed suggest possible diagnoses of polycystic ovaries, late-onset adrenal hyperplasia (LOAH), or both (as the two conditions coexist in 10–15% of cases). The latter is diagnosed by Synacthen testing (ACTH 250 μg intravenously), and measure levels of cortisol, androstenedione and 17-hydroxyprogesterone at time 0, 30 and 60 minutes (New *et al*, 1983; Azziz and Zacur, 1989). Unfortunately in this case ACTH was contraindicated because the patient had asthma, but the baseline levels were such that she must have had adrenal enzyme dysfunction which led to an accumulation of 17-hydroxyprogesterone (**Q5**).

All the statements concerning 17-hydroxyprogesterone are true. It is therefore very important to standardize measurement of this precursor in order to enable correct interpretation. 17-Hydroxyprogesterone should be measured at 0900 hours on days 5–15 of the menstrual cycle. The same should be applied to the measurement of other hormone, particularly LH (**Q6**).

Clomiphene citrate is a serum oestrogen receptor modulator drug type and used to be known as an antioestrogen. It is a very simple, cheap and effective way of overcoming infrequent ovulation. The multiple pregnancy rate with its use is approximately 10%, the vast majority of which will be dizygotic twins. It is indicated in women with chronic anovulation for most causes except hyperprolactinaemia, thyroid dysfunction, and hypogonadotrophic and hypergonadotrophic hypogonadism. A common side-effect is headache and the maximum recommended dose is 250 mg per day in the follicular phase of the cycle, usually days 2–6. Many clinicians would limit its use to 100 mg per day (**Q7: true = A, D; false = B, C, E**).

There were two alternative methods of ovulation induction at this stage: pure FSH or the combination of FSH–LH (HMG). In this case it would seem reasonable, with the raised level of serum LH, to recommend pure FSH

(**Q8**). It is not surprising that the ovaries were hyperstimulated. The best way to manage this patient would have been to correct the identified endocrinopathy, i.e. to suppress the mild adrenal enzyme dysfunction and normalize hormonal levels before proceeding to induction of ovulation.

Stimulated cycles must be monitored with ultrasound scans and possibly oestradiol estimations. Patients must be made aware of the potential risks of hyperstimulation, including the increased rate of multiple pregnancy. Admission to hospital must be available if ovarian hyperstimulation syndrome develops and experienced clinicians must be available to deal with this potentially serious complication. There is a theoretical increased risk of ovarian cancer with recurrent use of agents that induce ovulation (**Q9**).

The aim with FSH administration is to develop follicles to or in excess of 16 mm in diameter with as little FSH as possible. The oestradiol levels were satisfactory (500–1000 pmol l^{-1} per follicle). At this stage the best option was to 'coast' or to give no more FSH and watch the follicular growth (**Q10**).

Assuming this woman has an inherited disorder of adrenal enzyme function (LOAH) and the prevalence of total 21-hydroxylase deficiency (classical congenital adrenal hyperplasia) in the community is about 1 in 35, it is important to continue treatment until sexual development of the fetus is complete, especially if the fetus is a female. The fetus may be at risk of masculinization *in utero* if it has inherited two abnormal 21-hydroxylase activity genes. Dexamethasone must be continued until 20 weeks' gestation and then slowly withdrawn over 2 weeks to allay the adrenal suppression that has been enforced by the dexamethasone.

REFERENCES

Azziz R, Zacur HA. 21-Hydroxylase deficiency in female hyperandrogenism: screening and diagnosis. *J Clin Endocrinol Metab* 1989; **69:** 577–584.

Ferriman D, Gallwey JD. Clinical assessment of hair growth in women. *J Clin Endocrinol* 1961; **21**: 1440–1447.

New MI, Lorenzen F, Lerner AJ et al. Genotyping steroid 21-hydroxylase deficiency: hormonal reference data. *J Clin Endocrinol Metab* 1983; **57**: 320–326.

FACTS YOU SHOULD HAVE LEARNT . . .

▶ The differential diagnosis and investigation of oligomenorrhoea
▶ The indications for and complications of clomiphene citrate therapy
▶ The principles regarding the use of gonadotrophins to induce ovulation

CASE 31

Dyspareunia and dysmenorrhoea

A 24-year-old P0+0 Caucasian woman had always had painful periods, but they had become worse over the previous 6 months. The pain started about 3 days before each period and reached its greatest intensity on the first day of bleeding. In addition, she had experienced a similar pain, although less severe, intermittently throughout the last three cycles. The periods were not particularly heavy and she had no other bleeding. She had experienced deep dyspareunia for several months. She had taken the oral contraception pill until 12 months before, but had not used any contraception since, in the hope of conceiving.

Q1: **Which of the following should the differential diagnosis include?**
A: Fibroids.
B: Pelvic venous congestion.
C: Carcinoma of the endometrium.
D: Endometriosis.

Abdominal examination was unremarkable, but pelvic assessment revealed a retroverted and tender uterus with an 'orange-sized' mass in the left fornix.

Q2: **Which of the following investigations should you perform?**
A: A CA125 assay.
B: A hysterosalpingogram.
C: Fine-needle aspiration.
D: A pelvic ultrasound scan.

The patient was found to have an 8-cm mass arising from the left ovary following investigation. The uterus was retroverted but not enlarged, and the endometrium was not thickened.

Q3: **Which of the following should be included in your management plan?**
A: Danazol treatment for 6 months.
B: Laparoscopy with aspiration of the cyst.
C: Laparotomy with cystectomy or oöphorectomy.
D: Pelvic clearance.

At operation, a fixed tubo-ovarian mass was found on the left side of the uterus, with the latter stuck down in front of the rectum. The right adnexa was fairly normal with no adhesions and just some small spots of endometriosis on the right ovary. The left-sided mass was approached retroperitoneally by opening up the parietal peritoneum between the round ligament and ovarian vessels on the pelvic side wall. The left ureter was identified and avoided whilst freeing up the left tubo-ovarian mass. There was no residual ovarian tissue outside the cyst wall and a left salpingo-oöphorectomy was performed. The uterus was mobilized posteriorly and the pelvis washed out with warm saline. The endometriotic deposits on the right ovary were destroyed with diathermy.

The patient made a good recovery and was discharged home 5 days later. Histological examination of the ovary confirmed an endometriotic cyst with no atypical epithelium.

Q4: How would you manage the patient now?

Over the following 6 months, her periods improved with very little pain and the dyspareunia was also much better. Unfortunately, she failed to conceive, and she and her husband requested investigation for infertility. Her hormonal profile was normal and a mid-luteal phase progesterone level was well into the ovulatory range. Her husband's semen analysis was normal. It was decided to perform a laparoscopy with dye studies. Nine months had elapsed since the laparotomy.

At operation, the right tube and ovary were free and there was fill and spill of dye through the right tube. There were some small endometriotic deposits on the uterosacral ligaments.

Q5: Which of the following should be included in your management plan?
A: Danazol treatment.
B: In vitro assisted reproduction techniques.
C: Falloposcopy.
D: Reassurance.

After informed counselling, the couple decided to do nothing further for 12 months in the hope that spontaneous conception would occur. Unfortunately this did not happen and gradually the woman's periods became more painful and the dyspareunia recurred. Pelvic assessment revealed a retroverted immobile uterus with a tender nodule in the pouch of Douglas. The couple were becoming very depressed at their failure to conceive and wished to consider in vitro fertilization.

Q6: How would you counsel them?

In spite of the risks of in vitro fertilization, the couple opted to pursue this option. During the first cycle of treatment, the woman experienced severe lower abdominal pain mid-cycle and was admitted as an emergency. An ultrasound scan revealed a 6 cm ovarian cyst with free fluid in the pouch of Douglas.

Q7: Which of the following should be included in your management plan?

A: Intravenous fluids and analgesics.

B: Laparoscopy and drainage of the cyst.

C: Laparotomy.

Q8: What is your diagnosis and what are the complications of this condition?

The patient made a good recovery and a scan 1 week later revealed a normal right ovary.

It was decided to resume ovulation induction and *in vitro* fertilization in the following cycle. The patient experienced much less pain, and fertilization with embryo transfer was achieved. A rising human chorionic gonadotrophin titre was recorded within 2 weeks. An ultrasound scan at 6 weeks confirmed an intrauterine twin gestation and the pregnancy progressed to the vaginal delivery of two healthy male infants at 38 weeks' gestation.

COMMENTARY

In a patient presenting with such symptoms, the most likely diagnosis is endometriosis, although pelvic venous congestion is a possibility. Fibroids usually cause menorrhagia with pain commencing at the start of the period. Endometrial cancer presents with irregular bleeding, and is extremely rare under the age of 40 years (**Q1: true = B, D; false = A, C**). The presence of a mass on vaginal examination would exclude pelvic congestion, and the most useful investigation would be a pelvic ultrasound scan. This may reveal altered blood within the cyst. While use of the CA125 assay is widely recognized in epithelial ovarian cancer, it is the most useful diagnostic marker for endometriosis (Pittaway and Douglas, 1989). Hysterosalpingography and fine-needle aspiration would not be appropriate investigations, as neither will affect subsequent management (**Q2: true = A, D; false = B, C**).

Endometriosis may be managed medically or surgically. The rationale behind medical treatment is ovarian suppression resulting in resolution of the disease over a period of 6–9 months. In this case, the use of drugs is unlikely to cause the cyst to disappear and surgical management would be advisable. A laparoscopy with cyst aspiration would not be therapeutic as active disease would remain, and the patient should undergo laparotomy with removal of the cyst, possibly necessitating oöphorectomy. Whilst pelvic clearance is the definitive treatment for severe endometriosis, you should be very reluctant to recommend this in a 24-year-old nulliparous patient. In addition to dealing with the cyst, a laparotomy will allow adhesiolysis and destruction of small endometriotic deposits. Only surgeons with considerable skill and experience in minimal access surgery would advocate such an approach in this patient (**Q3: true = C; false = A, B, D**).

Following surgery, you have to decide whether to administer drug treatment to suppress the endometriosis. In this case, it has been adequately dealt with at operation and, even if there is a small amount of disease remaining, there is no evidence that medical treatment will benefit the patient, particularly from the point of view of fertility (Thomas and Cooke, 1987). Indeed, such therapy will delay the woman the opportunity to conceive. If she does become pregnant, this is an excellent treatment for endometriosis. On balance, the authors would not give any further treatment at this stage, and in fact her symptoms subsequently improved (**Q4**).

After the laparoscopy with dye studies, there were some small endometriotic deposits on the uterosacral ligaments. There would be no reason to treat the endometriosis at this stage, as it is asymptomatic and treatment will not improve fertility. With regard to her failure to conceive, there is no evidence of ovulation failure or poor sperm production, and, if anything, the only possible problem is one of transport. Whilst the right tube is patent, there may be intrinsic damage possibly related to retrograde menstruation and active endometriosis in the past. It would be reasonable to perform a falloposcopy to assess the lumen, but equally acceptable to do nothing further at this stage as the patient has been off the oral contraceptive pill for less than 2 years and it is only 9 months since the laparotomy. It is probably too early to consider *in vitro* fertilization (**Q5: true = C, D; false = A, B**).

Twelve months later, she has not conceived and the endometriosis is clearly becoming more active again. She ought to receive treatment to suppress it, but this will delay her chance to conceive. To proceed to *in vitro* fertilization, it will be necessary to induce ovulation and this may well stimulate the disease, with worsening symptoms. In counselling the couple, the options are either to try to achieve pregnancy with three cycles of *in vitro* fertilization, or to suppress ovarian activity with high-dose progestogen or danazol for 6 months and then proceed to *in vitro* fertilization. The authors favour the latter approach, although in this case the couple opted for immediate assisted conception (**Q6**).

During the first cycle of treatment, the woman developed ovarian hyperstimulation syndrome with a 6 cm cyst. Management should be conservative and supportive with fluids and analgesia. Surgery is not appropriate unless there is evidence of peritonitis (**Q7: true = A; false = B, C**). The condition is usually self-resolving, although it can occasionally be very serious. Electrolyte imbalances can occur and the patient may develop heart failure and adult respiratory distress syndrome, which may be fatal. The risks are greater with the use of gonadotrophin therapy. Another possibly serious consequence of ovulation induction is a long-term increase in the risk of developing ovarian cancer (Spirtas *et al*, 1993) (**Q8**).

REFERENCES

Pittaway DE, Douglas JW. Serum CA-125 in women with endometriosis and chronic pelvic pain. *Fertil Steril* 1989; **51**: 68–70.

Spirtas R, Kaufman SC, Alexander NJ. Fertility drugs and ovarian cancer – red alert or red herring? *Fertil Steril* 1993; **59**: 291–293.

Thomas EJ, Cooke ID. Successful treatment of asymptomatic endometriosis: does it benefit infertile women? *BMJ* 1987; **294**: 117–119.

FACTS YOU SHOULD HAVE LEARNT . . .

▶ The surgical management of endometriosis
▶ The relationship between endometriosis and fertility
▶ The investigation, complications and management of ovarian hyperstimulation syndrome

CASE 32

Dysfunctional uterine bleeding

A 32-year-old Caucasian woman presented with a 6-month history of increasingly heavy periods. Her menstrual cycle was regular, every 28 days, with bleeding lasting for 6 days. The loss was very heavy for 3 days with the passage of large blood clots and it gradually settled over the final 3 days. She experienced some lower abdominal discomfort when the bleeding was heavy, although she did not need to take analgesics. There was no mid-cycle or postcoital bleeding and she had had a recent negative smear. She had two children, both delivered normally, and used a diaphragm for contraception. Abdominal examination was unremarkable and vaginal assessment revealed a healthy cervix, a fully mobile anteverted uterus and no other pelvic mass.

Q1:   Which of the following would be appropriate management options?
A: Hysterectomy.
B: Administration of mefenamic acid.
C: Administration of buserelin.
D: Diagnostic curettage.
E: Administration of tranexamic acid.

The haemoglobin concentration was $11.0 \, \mathrm{g \, dl^{-1}}$. After discussing the management options, the patient was advised to take tranexamic acid 1 g four times per day during her menstrual periods. She was to be reviewed in 3 months' time.

At the next visit, her symptoms were unchanged. She was keen not to take any more medication.

Q2:   How would you counsel her regarding further management?

She considered that a hysterectomy was too radical at her age even though she did not wish to have any more children. She decided that she would undergo an endometrial resection. A date for surgery was arranged for 2 months later and she was advised to take danazol 200 mg three times per day for 4 weeks before surgery. An ultrasound scan showed a normal uterine cavity.

Q3:   Which of the following are side effects of danazol?
A: Visual disturbance.
B: Tinnitus.
C: Irreversible deepening of the voice.
D: Hirsutism.
E: Leucopenia.

After taking the danazol for 1 week, the woman was unable to tolerate the side-effects. She reported to the outpatient clinic, where she was given a subcutaneous injection of goserelin (3.6 mg).

She underwent a laparoscopic sterilization and transcervical endometrial resection 3 weeks later. The uterine cornua and the fundus was treated with the diathermy rollerball, with the remaining endometrium was removed with the diathermy loop to the level of the internal cervical os.

Q4: What are the immediate complications of endometrial resection and what precautions would you take to avoid them?

The patient went home the following day and was given an outpatient appointment for 3 months later. After the operation she bled for 4 weeks, although the flow was not heavy, and it became more of a brown discharge after the first 2 weeks. She had no further bleeding before the outpatient attendance. She was discharged from the clinic on that occasion.

Six months later, she was referred back with severe cyclical pain for 2 days every 4 weeks. It was suprapubic and she described it as a cramp. She had not had any vaginal bleeding.

Q5: What is the problem and how would you deal with it?

Hysteroscopic examination of the uterine cavity revealed synechiae between the anterior and posterior walls. It was possible to divide these with the hysteroscope and at the end of the procedure a multiload copper 250 coil was left in the uterus.

The coil was removed 3 months later, but unfortunately the pain returned within 3 months although she continued to be amenorrhoeic.

Q6: Which of the following treatment options would you recommend?
A: Repeat endometrial resection.
B: Administration of the oral contraceptive pill.
C: Administration of mefenamic acid.
D: Hysterectomy.

The patient elected to undergo hysterectomy. At the time of the endometrial resection, there was no significant uterine prolapse and the hysterectomy was carried out via the abdominal route. The ovaries were conserved.

Q7: Which of the following are complications of hysterectomy?
A: Lymphocyst formation.
B: Premature menopause.
C: Internal iliac artery aneurysm.
D: Uterovaginal fistula.
E: Irritable bowel syndrome.

The operation was uncomplicated and the patient made a good recovery. When she was seen 2 months later, the pain had completely resolved. She was discharged from the clinic.

COMMENTARY

The majority of cases of abnormal premenopausal bleeding are due to dysfunctional bleeding. In a 32-year-old woman with menorrhagia and completely regular cycles, the possible other causes include fibroids, endometriosis and the use of an intrauterine contraceptive device. In the case described, these were effectively excluded at the initial consultation. Whilst all the suggested options are of potential benefit, except diagnostic curettage, one would recommend non-hormonal medical therapy in the first instance. Tranexamic acid has been found to be the most effective therapy in reducing menstrual blood loss (Milsom *et al*, 1991), but was not helpful in this case (**Q1: true = B, E; false = A, C, D**). Other medical therapies, both non-hormonal or hormonal, could be tried next, although with the patient's reluctance to take further medication, you should counsel her regarding other options. Although the intrauterine progestagen delivery system is not licensed for the treatment of menorrhagia, its use in this situation is increasingly being advocated. Surgical treatments include destruction or removal of the endometrium with an operating hysteroscope, or hysterectomy. The advantages of the former include a less invasive procedure, shorter hospital stay and more rapid resumption of normal activities. There are, however, doubts about the long-term effectiveness of these procedures, whereas hysterectomy is guaranteed to cure the problem. You should also discuss the various types of hysterectomy, in particular the reduced morbidity of vaginal hysterectomy (**Q2**).

The results of endometrial destruction or resection are improved by preoperative endometrial preparation. The most widely used products are danazol and luteinizing hormone releasing hormone (LHRH) agonists, which have the effect of thinning the endometrium. Danazol has multiple side-effects, of which the most important are androgenic effects, abnormal bleeding, leucopenia, thrombocytopenia, visual disturbances, benign intracranial hypertension and cholestatic jaundice. LHRH analogues may produce menopausal symptoms, abnormal bleeding, depression, breast and ovarian cysts, blurred vision and a decrease in trabecular bone density (**Q3: true = A, C, D, E; false = B**).

When performing endometrial ablation or resection, you must inform the patient that further pregnancy should not be contemplated because of the risks of abnormal implantation and fetal malformation. Many women elect to be sterilized at the time of surgery and this may have the added advantage of reducing the amount of systemic absorption of the irrigating fluid. The immediate complications of endometrial resection include excessive and uncontrollable bleeding which may necessitate hysterectomy on rare occasions. The patient must be aware of this before surgery. Uterine perforation may occur at the time of the operation and, if not recognized, can have catastrophic consequences with damage to bladder, bowel and major vessels. The other main perioperative complication is absorption into the circulation of large amounts of glycine. This can result in fluid overload, haemolysis and hyponatraemia. A significant fall in the sodium level is associated with absorption of more than 1 litre of glycine (Bammann *et al*, 1990), and it is of paramount importance that the balance of irrigating fluid is closely monitored during the procedure. A deficit of more than 1 litre is regarded as an indication for immediate cessation of surgery (**Q4**).

In the longer term, endometrial resection may not be effective in reducing menstrual flow, with gradual regeneration of the endometrium. One of the risks of this procedure is the formation of intrauterine adhesions, resulting in complete amenorrhoea due to Asherman's syndrome. This may cause considerable pain as occurred in this case. The treatment options are either hysteroscopic exploration of the uterine cavity with breakdown of the adhesions and then insertion of an intrauterine contraceptive device (IUCD) to try to prevent adhesion recurrence, or hysterectomy (**Q5**). Oestrogen treatment should not be prescribed as, by stimulating the development of any remaining endometrium, there is a risk of recurrent menorrhagia. If hysteroscopic division of adhesions and IUCD insertion fails, the only cure is to perform a hysterectomy (**Q6: true = D; false = A, B, C**). This patient underwent hysterectomy, which is usually uncomplicated in a young woman with a mobile uterus. However, it can be associated with serious complications including urinary tract injury and fistula formation. In addition, it appears that ovarian failure occurs earlier in patients who have undergone hysterectomy and therefore premature menopause may occur (Siddle *et al*, 1987) (**Q7: true = B, D; false = A, C, E**).

REFERENCES

Bammann R, Magos AL, Kay JDS, Turnbull AC. Absorption of glycine irrigating solution during transcervical resection of endometrium. *BMJ* 1990, **300**: 304–305.

Milsom I, Andersson JK, Andersch B, Rybo G. A comparison of fluriprofen, tranexamic acid, and a levonorgestrel-releasing intrauterine contraceptive device in the treatment of idiopathic menorrhagia. *Am J Obstet Gynecol* 1991; **164**: 879–883.

Siddle N, Sarrel L, Whitehead M. The effect of hysterectomy on the age at ovarian failure. *Fertil Steril* 1987; **47**: 94–100.

FACTS YOU SHOULD HAVE LEARNT . . .

- ▶ The options for treating menorrhagia
- ▶ The indications for and complications of endometrial resection
- ▶ The complications of hysterectomy

CASE 33

Menorrhagia with uterine enlargement

A 28-year-old single nulligravida Caucasian solicitor was referred to the gynaecology clinic with a 3-year history of increasingly heavy periods. She had sought the advice of her general practitioner, who had prescribed norethisterone 5 mg three times daily with no good effect.

QI: Which of the following statements about norethisterone are correct?

A: It is a 19-carbon atom containing synthetic progestogen derived from testosterone.

B: It is a 21-carbon atom containing naturally occurring progesterone.

C: In the UK 40% of women receiving medical treatment for menorrhagia are prescribed norethisterone.

D: Norethisterone has been found to be no more effective than placebo in the short-term treatment of menorrhagia.

E: Norethisterone should no longer be prescribed for the medical treatment of menorrhagia.

Her menarche had been at the age of 14 years and her periods had always been regular, lasting 3–4 days every 26–28 days. She had had a recent normal cervical smear and did not complain of any intermenstrual bleeding. She was in a homosexual relationship and gave no obvious history to suggest previous pelvic infection. Over the preceding 2 years she had noticed increasing dysmenorrhoea lasting for 2 days. The heaviness of her menstrual flow meant that she regularly missed 1 or 2 days of work most months and that she soiled her bedclothes despite wearing double protection. To her knowledge she had not been anaemic and had not suffered any other medical or surgical illnesses. She was a non-smoker. She had never practised any form of contraception. She had no gastrointestinal symptoms.

Q2:   Explain the differences between menorrhagia, heavy periods and dysfunctional uterine bleeding (DUB).

On examination the patient looked slightly pale but otherwise well. There was no goitre, her breasts were normal and abdominal palpation was normal with no masses found. Pelvic examination revealed a normal-looking vagina and cervix. The uterus was anteverted, mobile, tender and uniformly enlarged, approximately equal to an 8-week gravid uterus. There were no pelvic masses or uterosacral nodularity and the adnexae were not tender.

Q3: Which of the following conditions can cause uterine tenderness?
  A: Endometrial hyperplasia with severe architectural and cytological atypia.
  B: Endometritis.
  C: Salpingitis isthmica nodosa.
  D: Adenomyosis uteri.
  E: Fibromas.
  F: Endometriosis.

A full blood count revealed a haemoglobin concentration of 9.9 g dl^{-1} with a low mean cell volume (MCV) of 69.0 fl and a low mean cell haemoglobin (MCH) of 24 pg, but other parameters were normal. Thyroid function was normal and a day 19 endometrial biopsy revealed secretory endometrium.

Q4: What conclusions do you draw from these results?

Q5: What medical treatment options are available?

A pelvic ultrasound scan was arranged and the uterus was imaged (Figure 3):

Q6: How would you describe the scan and what is the differential diagnosis?

Q7: What are the surgical options available for this woman?

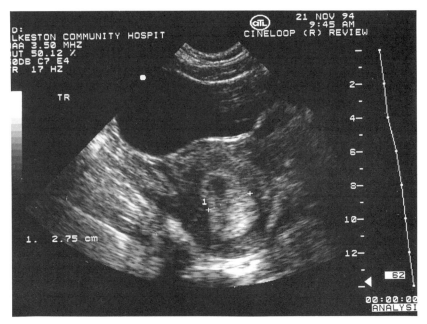

Figure 3   Transvaginal ultrasonography of the uterus.

Following detailed discussions she decided to have an abdominal hysterectomy with ovarian conservation. This was performed without complication and there was no evidence of peritoneal or ovarian endometriosis or previous pelvic inflammatory disease.

Q8: What are the complications associated with abdominal hysterectomy?

The histology revealed a large adenomyoma but was otherwise normal.

Q9: Which of the following statements concerning adenomyosis are true?
   A: Adenomyosis is the presence of endometrial glandular structures within the myometrium.
   B: Concomitant endometriosis is found in 10–20% of cases of adenomyosis at hysterectomy.
   C: Adenomyosis has a strong positive correlation with parity and is very rare in nulliparous women.
   D: All cases of adenomyosis are symptomatic.
   E: Imaging techniques have a sensitivity and specificity of around 80% in the diagnosis of adenomyosis.

Q10: What are the advantages and disadvantages of endometrial resection or ablation over hysterectomy for women with heavy periods?

COMMENTARY

The majority of the following information concerning menorrhagia comes from the bulletin *Effective Health Care* (1995). This document is essential reading for trainees in obstetrics and gynaecology.

Norethisterone is a 19-carbon atom, steroid ring structure, synthetic progestogen that is derived from testosterone and thus has androgenic effects and side-effects. In current medical practice in the UK nearly 40% of women receiving medical treatment for menorrhagia are prescribed norethisterone and it is true that it has been found to be no more effective than placebo in the short-term treatment of menorrhagia. However, it is efficacious in women with anovulatory menorrhagia (**Q1: true = A, C, D; false = B, E**).

Menorrhagia is an 'excessive' regular menstrual blood loss. 'Excessive' is objectively defined as menstrual blood loss greater than 80 ml as recorded by techniques. This figure was obtained from population studies where the mean blood loss was 30–40 ml and 90% of women had a smaller loss than 80 ml. However, estimation of blood loss is not feasible in current routine clinical practice. Heavy periods is a subjective symptom; approximately 30% of women who seek medical treatment do not actually have loss greater than average. You are obliged to ascertain from the history the degree of blood loss and its effect on the quality of life. Indirect objective evidence should be sought to support the syptomatology. This includes evidence of anaemia and iron deficiency (e.g. low MCH and/or MCV on a full blood count). Dysfunctional uterine bleeding (DUB) is a collective term to describe a condition where the clinician has failed to find a cause for heavy periods. DUB should really be described as ovulatory menorrhagia (**Q2**).

The conditions that can cause uterine tenderness on examination include endometritis, adenomyosis, fibroids and endometriosis (if the endometriosis involves the uterus and surrounding peritoneal structures). Endometriosis is present in approximately 10–20% of cases of adenomyosis. Endometrial hyperplasia with severe architectural and cytological atypia and salpingitis isthmica nodosa are not associated with uterine tenderness. Uterine tenderness is an important physical sign that, when elicited, should alert you to the above-mentioned diagnoses (**Q3: true = B, D, E, F; false = A, C**).

The results show an iron deficiency picture which supports the patient's claim of heavy periods in that she was probably losing more iron than she consumed each month. The patient therefore requires a haematinic agent to redress that imbalance. The fact that secretory endometrium was obtained confirms ovulation (**Q4**). Antifibrinolytic drugs, non-steroidal anti-inflammatory agents or an intrauterine progestogen delivery system should be considered if uterine causes have been excluded (**Q5**).

There is a large ill-defined echogenic region adjacent to the endometrial cavity with uterine enlargement. The differential diagnosis includes fibroids, adenomyosis or possibly a tumour. It would be possible to perform a directed biopsy of the myometrium to confirm the diagnosis (Popp *et al*, 1993). The distinction could also be made with a trial of pituitary down-regulation using a gonadotrophin releasing hormone analogue; a fibroid would regress but an adenomyoma would not. The latter option would have the added advantage of reducing blood loss and would help by improving the haemoglobin concentration (**Q6**).

The surgical options available for this woman include hysterectomy if fertility does not need to be preserved or myomectomy if the lesion is proved to be a fibroid. Endometrial resection is not a preferred option in this situation as the patient's dysmenorrhoea will not be treated. She must understand that a hysterectomy will render her sterile, necessitate 2–3 months' convalescence, is curative and has a high level of satisfaction. The procedure has a mortality rate of between 0.4 and 2 per 1000 women and an overall postoperative complication rate of 45%. Hysterectomy has been implicated in long-term conditions such as bowel disorder, urinary symptoms, osteoarthritis, earlier menopause and a reduction in cervical orgasm (**Q7**).

When discussing postoperative complications, your answer should have some structure, for example intraoperative, perioperative, short-term postoperative and long-term postoperative complications. The complications associated with abdominal hysterectomy include pain, haemorrhage, wound infection, urinary retention, urine infection and venous thromboembolism. Many measures can be instituted to help reduce these risks, including preoperative antibiotic prophylaxis, thromboprophylaxis, early mobilization, and care and attention to sterile techniques when performing urinary catheterization (**Q8**).

Adenomyosis is the presence of endometrial glandular and stromal structures within the myometrium and of myometrial hyperplasia. Concomitant endometriosis is found in 10–20% of cases of adenomyosis and has a strong positive correlation with parity but is not rare in nulliparous women (5–10%), as in this case. Not all cases of adenomyosis are symptomatic. Imaging techniques like vaginal ultrasonography and magnetic resonance imaging seem to have a sensitivity and specificity in the order of 80% in the diagnosis of adenomyosis (**Q9: true = B, E; false = A, C, D**).

Endometrial resection or ablation generally results in a shorter operating time with a lower postoperative complication rate than hysterectomy. Women require a shorter period in hospital and they resume normal activities earlier than those who have undergone hysterectomy. There appear to be cost benefits but these must be offset against the need to perform a hysterectomy in 23% of cases within 2 years. The long-term effects of endometrial resection or ablation remain unknown. Endometrial resection or ablation is not always successful in reducing menstrual loss, and dysmenorrhoea may increase. Initial patient satisfaction appears to disappear 4 months after the operation. Vaginal hysterectomy has fewer complications and a shorter hospital stay, and is less costly than abdominal hysterectomy. Laparoscopically assigned vaginal hysterectomy is a possible alternative that remains to be evaluated in terms of clinical and cost effectiveness (**Q10**).

REFERENCES

The management of menorrhagia. University of Leeds. Churchill Livingstone, Halifax. *Effective Health Care* 1995; **9**: 1–14.

Popp LW, Schweidessen JP, Gaetje R. Myometrial biopsy: its use in diagnosing adenomyosis uteri. *Am J Obstet Gynecol* 1993; **169**: 546–549.

FACTS YOU SHOULD HAVE LEARNT . . .

▶ **The definition of menorrhagia**
▶ **The differential diagnosis of menorrhagia and an enlarged uterus**
▶ **The management of adenomyosis**

CASE 34

Premenstrual syndrome

A 40-year-old woman presented to her general practitioner with vague symptoms of malaise, lethargy, lack of concentration, loss of libido and a general feeling of discontent. She worked part-time in a ladies fashion shop, was married to a successful businessman and had two healthy teenage children who were doing well at school. She had no other complaints although her menstrual periods were heavier than they had been in the past.

> **QI:** **Which of the following should be included in the differential diagnosis?**
> A: Hyperthyroidism.
> B: Premenstrual syndrome.
> C: Endogenous depression.
> D: Diabetes mellitus.
> E: Reactive depression.

On further questioning, it became apparent that she felt at her best towards the end of each period and for 1 week thereafter. Her symptoms then increased throughout the cycle and became maximal in the few days before menstruation. She took multivitamins regularly and had done so for a number of years. She did not use contraception as she had been sterilized shortly after her second child was born. She had no past history of depression. Her general practitioner thought that she had premenstrual syndrome. He advised her to take oil of evening primrose for a period of 3 months to see whether this helped her symptoms.

> **Q2:** **How would you describe and classify premenstrual syndrome?**

> **Q3:** **What is the aetiology of the syndrome?**

Unfortunately she did not gain much help from this treatment and the only new development before her next attendance was that her periods became more heavy and painful. The general practitioner performed a vaginal examination and found normal pelvic anatomy.

> **Q4:** **Which of the following management options would you recommend?**
> A: Referral for a specialist opinion.
> B: Hysterectomy.
> C: The combined oral contraceptive pill.
> D: Tricyclic antidepressants.
> E: Psychotherapy.

The patient had not smoked for about 5 years and her blood pressure was 130/80 mmHg. Her general practitioner suggested that, whilst she did not require contraception, the combined oral contraceptive pill might well improve her symptoms and she agreed to take Ovranette for a trial period of 3 months.

Q5: Why should the combined pill be helpful in premenstrual syndrome?

The contraceptive pill helped the periods from the point of view of pain and heavy menstrual bleeding. However, her other symptoms remained largely unchanged.

Q6: What other drug therapies may be of benefit?

Q7: Are there any other treatment options?

She did not wish to take any further hormonal preparations and the general practitioner decided to refer her to a gynaecologist for a further opinion.

After counselling, the patient did not consider that her symptoms justified any surgical intervention. With her unwillingness to use hormonal treatments, the gynaecologist did not have anything further to offer. He advised regular meals with boosts of carbohydrate throughout the day and suggested that she may like to attend a psychotherapist. The woman declined this, but she went to see a local homoeopath and also took some herbal treatment. This improved her symptoms for several months.

One year later she re-attended the general practitioner's surgery with her original symptoms intensified and associated with cyclical anxiety attacks, headaches and aggressive behaviour in the week before each period. The periods were regular and not particularly heavy. She thought she would like to see the gynaecologist again with a view to surgical treatment.

Q8: What, if any, surgical intervention would you advise?

She underwent a total abdominal hysterectomy and bilateral salpingo-oöphorectomy. The operation was an uncomplicated procedure and she recovered well. Six months later, she felt 'better than ever' and was using oestrogen skin patches for hormone replacement. She was discharged back to her general practitioner.

Q9: When would you have started hormone replacement therapy following surgery?

COMMENTARY

The presenting symptoms in this case may be due to a number of causes and it is necessary to probe further to try to be more precise. Hypothyroidism may be implicated, as may premenstrual syndrome and endogenous depression. There does not appear to be any cause for her reactive depression from the information given, and hyperthyroidism and diabetes mellitus do not present in this way (**Q1: true = B, C; false = A, D, E**).

Premenstrual syndrome may be defined as the cyclical recurrence of psychological, behavioural or somatic symptoms in the luteal phase of the menstrual cycle (O'Brien, 1987). It is a multifactorial condition, the diagnosis of which is more dependent on the timing of symptoms rather than their type. The fact that this woman's complaints occurred in the luteal phase of the cycle is highly suggestive of premenstrual syndrome. Apart from the timing of the symptoms, the syndrome may be classified according to symptom type, namely psychological, somatic or behavioural (**Q2**).

The precise aetiology of premenstrual syndrome is unknown but there are various hypothesis including the following:

▶ High oestrogen : progesterone ratio premenstrually.

▶ Premenstrual progesterone deficiency.

▶ Decreased sex hormone binding globulin.

▶ Hypoglycaemia.

▶ Fluid retention.

▶ Vitamin deficiency.

▶ Psychological factors.

▶ Genetic factors.   (**Q3**)

Numerous treatments have been tried, mainly aimed at the aetiological factors described above. It is probably most helpful to try to tailor treatments to particular symptoms, for example using diuretics for fluid retention and psychotherapy for psychological problems. In general, simple treatments such as vitamins are often tried initially. In the case described, after the option of oil of evening primrose had been unsuccessful, it was reasonable to use the oral contraceptive pill in view of her heavy periods (**Q4: true = C; false = A, B, D, E**). In fact, there is little good evidence supporting the effectiveness of the oral contraceptive pill in premenstrual syndrome. The Royal College of General Practitioners' (1974) study of 23 611 oral contraceptive takers and 22 766 controls found that users of the combined pill reported premenstrual syndrome 29% less commonly than those in the control group. Why the pill should be effective is uncertain. If ovulation is implicated in the aetiology as well as oestrogen and progesterone levels and ratios, then the pill will clearly affect all of these (**Q5**).

Other drugs that have been employed in premenstrual syndrome include progesterone and progestogens, oestradiol, danazol, bromocriptine, gonadotrophin releasing hormone analogues, inhibitors of prostaglandin, opiate antagonists, antidepressants and serotonin reuptake inhibitors (**Q6**). Apart from drugs, other therapies include counselling, psychotherapy, regular carbohydrate intake and various placebos (**Q7**).

In women with severe premenstrual syndrome unresponsive to other treatments, you may embark on surgical treatment. Removal of the ovaries has been found to be effective in this condition, although hysterectomy with ovarian conservation is generally not considered particularly useful. There is no point in leaving the uterus at the time of bilateral oöphorectomy, and in the case described hysterectomy would also have cured the menorrhagia (**Q8**).

Oestradiol treatment has been employed with some success in premenstrual syndrome and there would be no indication to withhold or delay hormone replacement following surgery in this case (**Q9**).

REFERENCES

O'Brien PMS. *The Pre-menstrual Syndrome*, pp 5–37. London: Blackwell Scientific Publications, 1987.

Royal College of General Practitioners. *Oral Contraception and Health*. London: Pittman Medical, 1974.

FACTS YOU SHOULD HAVE LEARNT . . .

▶ **The differential diagnosis of premenstrual syndrome**
▶ **The definition and classification of premenstrual syndrome**
▶ **The aetiology of premenstrual syndrome**
▶ **The management of premenstrual syndrome**

CASE 35

Uterine fibroids

A 27-year-old woman was referred to her local hospital with a history of increasingly heavy and painful menstrual periods over the preceding 2 years. Her cycles were regular with no intermenstrual bleeding and a recent cervical smear had been reported as negative. Her menstrual periods lasted for 7 days with very heavy loss for the first 2 days. The pain eased up after the second day. Apart from simple analgesics, she had not been given any treatment for the periods.

> **Q1: Which of the following should be included in the differential diagnosis?**
> A: Endometriosis.
> B: Pelvic infection.
> C: Uterine fibroids.
> D: Cervical ectropion.
> E: Endometrial carcinoma.

On further questioning, the patient was nulliparous and had used the oral contraceptive pill until 6 months before the consultation. She was not currently using any contraception. Whilst she was not actively trying to conceive, she did not mind whether she became pregnant.

On abdominal palpation, a firm pelvic mass was felt, reaching 5 cm above the symphysis pubis. On bimanual examination, the uterus was mobile with a size of approximately 16 weeks. It felt irregular. There were no other pelvic masses palpable.

> **Q2: What investigations would you perform?**

The haemoglobin level was 10 g dl^{-1} and a pelvic ultrasound scan confirmed an anterior wall fibroid 8 cm in diameter.

> **Q3: What are the treatment options?**

> **Q4: How would you counsel her regarding the risks of pregnancy?**

The patient was very keen to avoid surgery if at all possible, and she elected to try non-hormonal medical treatment initially. She was prescribed mefenamic acid 500 mg three times per day during her periods. A follow-up appointment was made for 3 months later.

At the follow-up visit, she had not had a period for 6 weeks and felt very tired. A pregnancy test was positive and an ultrasound scan showed a 5-week sized gestation sac in the uterus with no obvious fetal parts.

She was due to return for a further ultrasound scan 2 weeks later, but was admitted before that with heavy vaginal bleeding. Examination revealed an open cervix with blood clots in the vagina and she underwent evacuation for retained products. The histology report confirmed placental tissue. The haemoglobin level dropped to 8 g dl^{-1} and the patient was given iron supplementation. A follow-up appointment was made for her to be reviewed in a further 6 weeks' time.

When she was reviewed, she gave a history of one menstrual period which had been very heavy. She decided to continue using mefenamic acid for the menorrhagia. She was concerned that the fibroid may have caused the miscarriage.

Q5:   How would you counsel her regarding the miscarriage?

Three months later her periods were no better, and in view of the menorrhagia and the miscarriage, she decided to opt for a myomectomy. The fibroid was still 8 cm in diameter on an ultrasound scan.

Q6:   What are the risks of myomectomy?

Q7:   How would you try to minimize the risks?

As the patient was now quite keen to conceive, a date for surgery was arranged for 3 months hence. In the meantime, she received three subcutaneous injections of the gonadotrophin releasing hormone analogue goserelin, 3.6 mg at monthly intervals, in order to shrink the fibroid as much as possible before surgery.

At operation, the fibroid was found to be on the right side of the uterus, and was very close to the cornua. An incision was made over the fibroid, which was shelled out. The cavity was closed with figure of eight sutures using polyglactin. The uterine serosa was closed with a continuous locked number three polypropylene suture. Care was taken to avoid the right Fallopian tube. Blood loss was estimated at 500 ml, and no blood transfusion was given as the preoperative haemoglobin level was 12 g dl^{-1}.

The patient made a satisfactory recovery and was allowed home after 5 days.

Six weeks later, she was well and had had one period which was less heavy than previously. The periods remained acceptable over the following months, but she failed to conceive within 12 months of surgery.

Q8:   What investigations would you recommend?

A decision to perform a laparoscopy was taken and at laparoscopy, there were some fine omental adhesions over the uterine scar, but the uterus was mobile and dye spilled freely from each tube. The tubes and ovaries appeared normal with no adhesions or distortion. Two small fibroids, each less than 1 cm, were noted on the posterior wall of the uterus. Hysterosalpingography revealed a normal-shaped uterine cavity.

Further investigations confirmed that she was ovulating regularly and that her partner's semen analysis was satisfactory.

Q9: What would you do about the fibroids?

Unfortunately, she failed to conceive during the next year. Pelvic ultrasonography showed that the fibroids were no larger. It was not considered that the fibroids were relevant to her failure to conceive. In view of her subfertility, she elected to undergo three cycles of *in vitro* fertilization. Sadly, she did not conceive. However, her periods remained acceptable.

COMMENTARY

Regular, heavy and painful menstrual periods may be caused by both fibroids and endometriosis. The pain often precedes the bleeding in endometriosis, whereas the reverse is more common with fibroids. Pelvic infection may be associated with abnormal bleeding, but this is usually irregular. Bleeding associated with a cervical ectropion is most commonly postcoital, and endometrial carcinoma causes irregular bleeding as well as being extremely rare before the age of 40 years (**Q1: true = A, C; false = B, D, E**).

A uterus containing fibroids and enlarged to the size of a 16-week pregnancy would certainly explain this patient's symptoms. You should wish to investigate for anaemia, as well as ordering a pelvic ultrasound scan. The scan would exclude any ovarian pathology as well as assessing the number and size of the uterine fibroids (**Q2**).

Medical treatments, either hormonal or non-hormonal, are rarely effective in the control of menorrhagia when a large fibroid is present. However, in a young woman without children, hysterectomy is not usually an option and myomectomy carries certain potential risks necessitating careful consideration. Whilst mefanamic acid is less effective than other medical treatments for menorrhagia, the patient was also complaining of pain with her periods. The use of mefenamic acid was thus not unreasonable in the short term whilst she came to terms with the diagnosis and the likely ultimate treatment (**Q3**).

The fact that the patient was not using any contraception was important because of the risks of pregnancy in association with a large fibroid. Fibroids may cause problems with conception, either due to distortion of the uterine cavity interfering with implantation or because of tubal distortion impairing fertilization and transport. If pregnancy does occur, there is an increased risk of miscarriage or preterm labour. Fibroids may also undergo degeneration in pregnancy, causing severe pain, and may cause unstable lies necessitating Caesarean section. There are also risks of myomectomy and therefore a balance has to be struck between dealing with the fibroids before embarking on pregnancy or trying to complete one's family and then deal with the fibroids if necessary afterwards (**Q4**).

It is possible that this patient's fibroid may have been implicated in the miscarriage, although early miscarriage is extremely common in the absence of fibroids. However, this incident combined with her period problems was sufficient to sway her decision towards surgical intervention, which in the authors' opinion was reasonable. It is believed that removal of fibroids to decrease the risk of miscarriage should be performed only for submucous fibroids (Treffos, 1990) (**Q5**).

The main specific risk of myomectomy is haemorrhage, which can rarely be so severe that control is impossible without resorting to hysterectomy. You should usually quote the risk of this as being about 1%. Disadvantages of myomectomy compared with hysterectomy are that it is not guaranteed to cure the menorrhagia, and that further fibroids may subsequently develop. From the point of view of a woman who wishes to conceive, risks of myomectomy include adhesions and distortion of the tubes or uterine cavity, interfering with conception and implantation (**Q6**).

You must try to minimize bleeding at the time of surgery and the first step is to use agents to reduce the size of the fibroids. Gonadotrophin releasing hormone agonists have been shown to be effective in doing this (Gardner and Shaw, 1992). Intraoperative attention to haemostasis and avoiding damage, particularly to the uterine cornua, are both extremely important, and the risk of adhesion formation may be decreased by washing out the pelvis with dextran at the end of the procedure (**Q7**).

It is generally considered that the best chance of conception is within 6 months of surgery, and failure to become pregnant within 1 year should prompt investigation. Baseline tests of ovulation and sperm production are important. The most important investigations in this woman would be assessments of tubal patency, the shape of the uterine cavity, and the presence of adhesions causing possible tubal distortion or interfering with release of the ovum to the fimbriae (**Q8**). In this case the investigations were reassuring. Two small posterior wall fibroids not distorting the uterine cavity would not be a cause for concern or any immediate action. In the long term, the only worry would be that they may become much larger or that more fibroids may develop (**Q9**).

REFERENCES

Treffos PE. Uterine causes of early pregnancy failure In: Huisjes HJ, Lund T (eds) *Early Pregnancy Failure*, pp 114–147. Edinburgh: Churchill Livingstone, 1990.

Gardner RL, Shaw RW. GnRH agonists and blood loss at surgery. In: Shaw AW (ed.) *Advances in Reproductive Endocrinology: Uterine Fibroids*, pp 123–134. Parthenon Publishing, 1992.

FACTS YOU SHOULD HAVE LEARNT . . .

> ▶ The differential diagnosis of regular, heavy, menstrual bleeding
> ▶ The aetiology and investigation of menorrhagia
> ▶ The management of uterine fibroids
> ▶ The complications of myomectomy

CASE 36

Pelvic inflammatory disease

A 33-year-old P3 + 3 West Indian woman was referred to a consultant gynaecologist with an 8-month history of pelvic pain which she described as 'a pain in her womb'. She also complained of a vaginal discharge which had improved following a course of antibiotics. Her menstrual history was normal and there was no history of amenorrhoea, dysmenorrhoea or dyspareunia.

> **Q1:** **What is the likely diagnosis at this early stage of the consultation?**
> A: Endometriosis.
> B: Pelvic inflammatory disease.
> C: Bacterial vaginosis.
> D: Colposamorosis fugax.
> E: Vulvodynia.

Her past medical history revealed a 5-year history of right upper quadrant pain which had remained undiagnosed despite gastroscopy and ultrasound scans of the kidneys, liver and gallbladder under the care of a consultant surgeon. She had been referred to a rheumatologist and a radiograph of the thoracic spine was normal. Haemoglobin electrophoresis was normal and hepatitis B surface antigen was positive although liver function was normal.

> **Q2:** **Do you think this past history is relevant other than in excluding a host of upper abdominal diagnoses?**

Recently she had separated from her boyfriend as he had been socializing with another woman. On examination, her body mass index was 25 kg m^{-2} and urinalysis was normal. She was tender in the right upper quadrant and in the suprapubic region. Vaginal examination revealed a healthy cervix with no discharge. The uterus was tender and retroverted and there was tenderness in the pouch of Douglas. There were no pelvic masses.

> **Q3:** **Which of the following signs and symptoms might support a diagnosis of pelvic inflammatory disease?**
> A: Metrorrhagia.
> B: Vaginal discharge.
> C: Dysuria.
> D: Pain of more than 9 days' duration.
> E: Fever greater than 38°C.

Q4: Which of the following investigations may be helpful?
A: Serum antichlamydial antibodies.
B: Full blood count, erythrocyte sedimentation rate, liver function tests.
C: Mid-stream urine for culture.
D: High vaginal swab for culture.
E: Endocervical swabs for culture.
F: Endometrial biopsy.

Q5: Are there any other investigations that you would perform?

As the patient had been recently treated with ampicillin and metronidazole by the general practitioner, she was prescribed oral doxycycline 100 mg twice daily for 14 days.

One month later she was admitted to hospital feeling unwell with abdominal pains and rigors, and a temperature of 38.8°C with a pulse rate of 90 beats per minute (bpm) and blood pressure of 140/80 mmHg. She was not vomiting but had anorexia. Her abdomen was tender but there were no signs of peritoneal irritation. Pelvic examination was essentially unchanged. All the investigations performed previously were negative or normal and the endometrial biopsy revealed secretory phase endometrium with no evidence of acute or chronic endometritis.

Q6: Which of the following should be included in the differential diagnosis?
A: Ectopic pregnancy.
B: Acute anorexia nervosa.
C: Septic abortion.
D: Salpingitis isthmica nodosa.
E: Pelvic inflammatory disease.

The patient was treated with bed rest, intravenous fluids and rectal metronidazole 1 g 8 hourly, doxycycline 100 mg orally 12 hourly and cefuroxime 750 mg intravenously every 6 hours. When she was reviewed by the genitourinary medicine consultant it was revealed that she had been a regular attender at the genitourinary medicine clinic over 15 years with several episodes of gonorrhoea and *Trichomonas vaginalis* infections. After 4 days of antibiotics, bed rest and intravenous fluids, the pain had resolved. Temperature and pulse rate were normal.

Q7: Would you consider diagnostic surgery at this stage?

A diagnostic laparoscopy was performed without complication. The pelvis was filled with fine new adhesions and a yellow thick gluey exudate was noted. The fimbrial ends of the Fallopian tubes were covered with the exudate and the ovaries appeared normal and relatively free of adhesions. The liver capsule was covered with fine 'violin string' adhesions and less taught, 'newer', adhesions which extended to the parietal peritoneum covering the inferior aspect of the right hemi-diaphragm. The fluid was aspirated and the pelvic cavity was washed out with normal saline.

Q8:   What is your diagnosis?

The postoperative course was uncomplicated and the patient was discharged on oral doxycycline 100 mg twice daily for a further week and indomethacin 100 mg three times daily as required.

Q9:   What advice would you give to this woman to avoid similar episodes of severe pelvic inflammatory disease?

Q10: What is the likely long-term prospect for this woman?

One month later she was reviewed in the outpatient clinic. She felt very well and was re-referred to the genitourinary medicine clinic for proof of cure, follow-up and contact tracing.

COMMENTARY

Whilst taking a history you should endeavour to obtain a diagnosis and then test your proposed diagnosis with the examination findings and investigations. At this stage the most likely diagnosis is pelvic inflammatory disease. Endometriosis can cause pelvic pain but usually leads to dysmenorrhoea and dyspareunia in symptomatic patients. Bacterial vaginosis does not, in itself, cause pelvic pain. Colposamorosis fugax does not exist and vulvodynia is vulval pain (**Q1: true = B; false = A, C, D, E**).

The history was very relevant and important for two reasons; firstly, you should have considered the diagnosis of perihepatitis or Fitz-Hugh–Curtis syndrome (Curtis, 1930; Fitz-Hugh, 1934), which is right upper abdominal pain and tenderness in a woman with pelvic inflammatory disease; secondly, the cause of the upper abdominal pain remained unknown. Perihepatitis occurs in up to 33% of women with salpingitis, and oral contraceptive use seems to reduce this incidence. *Neisseria gonorrhoeae* was thought to be the causative organism but most recent cases have been associated with *Chlamydia trachomatis* (**Q2**).

Intermenstrual bleeding and menorrhagia are more common with *Chlamydia*-associated pelvic inflammatory disease, and these symptoms are often associated with plasma cell endometritis. Young women, who are at high risk, are often overlooked and untreated, as plasma cell endometritis is very common. The presence of plasma cells in the endometrium is an objective test which helps to reduce the rate of false-negative laparoscopies for salpingitis (a subjective, operator-dependent test). Vaginal discharge is common and is often described as yellow and homogeneous. An offensive discharge is associated with trichomoniasis or bacterial vaginosis but is not necessarily characteristic of a diagnosis of pelvic inflammatory disease. Urinary frequency and dysuria are a consequence of urethritis, although these symptoms may be present in approximately 15–20% of cases of pelvic inflammatory disease. Pelvic pain is most commonly described as continuous, dull, gradual in onset, lower abdominal and often bilateral. The pain with gonorrhoea is probably more intense and patients seek medical advice within a few days, whereas chlamydial disease presents later. Fever is present in only about one-third of cases of pelvic inflammatory disease (**Q3: true = A, B, D, E; false = C**).

All the investigations could be performed but the most important are the endocervical swabs, especially for *N. gonorrhoeae* and *C. trachomatis*. An endometrial biopsy is a safe outpatient procedure and does not increase the infection rate. Chlamydial enzyme antigen detection tests are available and offer high sensitivity and specificity. The antigen detection tests overcome the difficulties of culturing this obligate intracellular organism, but commercially available kits are costly. *Chlamydia* infect the cells of the transformation zone of the cervix and adequate sampling of these cells is mandatory (at least 10 seconds is required to pick up the infected cells). The optimal microbiological diagnostic test must be arranged locally to maximize the detection rate and will depend on cost, transport and laboratory facilities. High vaginal swabs are only for diagnosing lower genital tract diseases such as vaginitis. Immunoglobulin (Ig) G and IgA serum antichlamydial antibodies are neither sensitive nor specific but have been used in the fertility clinic scenario as a discriminator to investigate tubal patency with either hysterosalpingography or laparoscopy. Leucocytosis and a raised erythrocyte sedimentation rate are related to the severity of the disease, and liver function tests are mandatory if perihepatitis is suspected (**Q4: true = A, B, C, D, E, F**).

An ultrasound scan may be helpful in the more severe cases especially to exclude ovarian cysts and pregnancy, and to confirm a pelvic abscess. The presence of an intrauterine viable pregnancy almost always precludes the diagnosis of pelvic inflammatory disease (**Q5**).

Pelvic inflammatory disease is the most likely diagnosis. Septic abortion and ectopic pregnancy would be excluded by a pregnancy test. The fact that all the results were negative previously does not exclude the diagnosis of pelvic inflammatory disease; the condition may have been only partially treated or re-infection may have occurred. Anorexia nervosa is an inappropriate diagnosis and salpingitis isthmica nodosa is an anatomical variant of the isthmus of the fallopian tube which consists of multiple channels through areas of muscle hypertrophy (**Q6: true = E, perhaps A, C; false = B, D**).

Surgery to establish a diagnosis is indicated in this case; the patient had been treated symptomatically thus far and the recent laboratory test results were not diagnostic. In addition, the right upper quadrant pain had remained undiagnosed for at least 6 years and the putative diagnosis of perihepatitis needed to be confirmed. The disadvantages of this option are the potential complications of anaesthesia and diagnostic laparoscopy, and the potential infective risk from hepatitis B for the surgeon, theatre staff and anaesthetist. These staff should have been immunized but good communication is important. Surgical double gown and gloves and protective glasses should be used (**Q7**).

The diagnosis of perihepatitis or Fitz-Hugh–Curtis syndrome has been confirmed along with pelvic inflammatory disease, in particular salpingitis (**Q8**).

This patient should be advised not to have sexual intercourse with her partner or partners unless they have been screened to diagnose and treat any sexually transmissible disease. She should never use an intrauterine device for contraception. Barrier methods and combined oral contraceptives offer the best protection against recurrent infection. The patient must be advised to seek advice early if her symptoms recur (**Q9**).

Unfortunately this patient is likely to become re-infected and to develop chronic debilitating pelvic pain (67% of patients with three or more episodes of pelvic inflammatory disease will have chronic pain), which seems to be related to the severity of the disease. Weight loss, general malaise and deterioration in her general health may occur and could require major pelvic surgery in the future with increased menstrual disturbance and dysmenorrhoea. She is at high risk of both ectopic pregnancy (the incidence after three or more episodes of pelvic inflammatory disease is 22%) and tubal infertility (the incidence after three or more episodes of pelvic inflammatory disease is 43%).

REFERENCES

Curtis AH. A cause of adhesions in the right upper quadrant. *JAMA* 1930; **94**: 1221–1222.

Fitz-Hugh T. Acute gonococcic peritonitis of the right upper quadrant in women. *JAMA* 1934; **102**: 2094–2096.

FACTS YOU SHOULD HAVE LEARNT . . .

> ▶ The signs and symptoms of pelvic inflammatory disease
> ▶ The appropriate investigations when pelvic inflammatory disease is suspected
> ▶ The sequelae of recurrent pelvic inflammatory disease

CASE 37

Pelvic abscess

A 21-year-old P0+0 Caucasian woman presented to the accident and emergency department with a 3-day history of increasing lower abdominal pain associated with vaginal bleeding. Her previous period had occurred 3 weeks earlier and had been normal. She had never had any abnormal bleeding before, and she took the oral contraceptive pill. The pain was colicky in nature and radiated around to her lower back. She had not gained any relief from simple analgesics.

On examination, she was flushed and looked unwell. She had a tachycardia of 110 beats per minute (bpm) and her temperature was 39°C. She was acutely tender across her lower abdomen with localized guarding. On vaginal assessment, there was some dark-coloured blood in the vagina. The cervix looked normal, but there was marked cervical excitation and it was impossible to outline the uterus or adnexa because of severe tenderness elicited when bimanual palpation was attempted.

> **Q1: Which of the following should be included in the differential diagnosis?**
> A: Pyelonephritis.
> B: Ectopic pregnancy.
> C: Complicated ovarian cyst.
> D: Appendicitis.
> E: Acute pelvic inflammatory disease.

> **Q2: What investigations would you perform?**

After establishing intravenous access, an infusion of Hartmann's solution was commenced and the patient was given doxycycline 100 mg intravenously to be repeated 12 hourly, and metronidazole 400 mg per rectum to be repeated 8 hourly.

A pregnancy test was negative, and the white cell count was raised at $22 \times 10^9 \, l^{-1}$. An ultrasound scan showed a complex mass arising in the region of the right ovary, 12 × 10 cm in size. The diagnosis of pelvic abscess was confirmed.

> **Q3. What are the management options?**

During the next 24 hours, her temperature fluctuated between 38 and 39°C. She required regular pethidine to control the pain and she was unable to tolerate oral fluids. The intravenous fluid regimen was maintained and the original antibiotic regimen was continued.

The erythrocyte sedimentation rate was 95. The swabs taken on admission were reported as follows:

- High vaginal swab – no growth.
- Cervical swab – *Chlamydia trachomatis* isolated.
- Urethral swab – *C. trachomatis* isolated.

It was decided to review the situation after a further 24 hours with an ultrasound scan.

Q4. Which of the following can result from a chlamydial infection?
A: Fitz-Hugh–Curtis syndrome.
B: Bartholin's abscess.
C: Reiter's disease.
D: Peripheral neuropathy.
E: Still's disease.

An ultrasound scan showed that the size of the pelvic collection was unchanged. The woman's clinical condition was much the same, with her temperature between 38 and 39°C and the need for analgesia unaltered.

Q5: How would you proceed?

The decision to operate was taken. It was impossible to identify the right tube and ovary, which were incorporated into the abscess. The left tube was buried in the pouch of Douglas with a normal-sized ovary just visible behind it. The uterus appeared to be normal in size, and was immobile and retroverted. The abscess cavity was drained and all the loculi and adhesions within it were broken down. The pelvis was washed out with warm saline and a large tube drain was inserted. The abdomen was closed.

The antibiotics were continued and the pus from the abscess grew *C. trachomatis*. She gradually recovered over the following few days and was allowed home after her temperature had settled for 48 hours and she was requiring only oral analgesics.

She was counselled about the need for contact tracing and was agreeable to this. She was referred to the local genitourinary medicine department and contact tracing was arranged.

Over the following 6 months, she complained of worsening and continuous pelvic discomfort which made intercourse impossible. She required increasingly strong analgesics to control the pain and to allow her to carry out normal activities. Examination revealed a fixed retroverted uterus with generalized tenderness.

Q6: Which of the following would you advise?
A: Pelvic clearance.
B: Referral to a pain specialist.
C: Laparoscopic adhesiolysis.
D: Continuous high-dose progestogen treatment.

After much discussion, a surgical option was agreed. A laparoscopy was performed; the findings were of a fixed uterus with multiple small bowel and peritoneal adhesions over it. The tubes and ovaries on either side were not visible. It was considered that an open adhesiolysis would be the safest option and this was performed. At the end of the procedure, it had been possible to free all the bowel adhesions and identify the ovaries, which were dissected off the uterus. The tubes were clearly non-functional on either side and the uterus remained relatively fixed.

Unfortunately, the chronic debilitating pain recurred over the following 4 months and the opinion of a pain specialist was sought. Various nerve blocks and epidural infusions were attempted with no suitable benefit, and the woman was referred back.

Q7: What options are now available?

Following prolonged counselling, the patient opted to undergo further surgery and a pelvic clearance was performed. She made a good recovery and was given oestrogen skin patches for hormone replacement. The pain was cured and she was able to return to normal activities.

COMMENTARY

The association of lower abdominal pain with abnormal vaginal bleeding is highly suggestive of a gynaecological problem, which is almost certainly infective with a temperature of 39°C and signs of a febrile illness. The likely diagnosis is acute pelvic inflammatory disease which may be complicated by an ovarian or tubal abscess (**Q1: true = C, E; false = A, B, D**).

In a situation of severe gynaecological infection, particularly in such a young woman, it is of paramount importance to isolate the responsible organism and instigate appropriate treatment to try to minimize any long-term damage. The most important investigations are cervical, urethral and high vaginal swabs, of which the first two are most likely to identify the most serious causes of pelvic infection, namely *C. trachomatis* and *Neisseria gonorrhoeae*. A raised white cell count confirms acute infection, and the erythrocyte sedimentation rate is often very high in pelvic inflammatory disease. It is worthwhile excluding pregnancy, particularly as tetracycline derivatives should be avoided in the first trimester. An ultrasound scan to look for an abscess is indicated when there are such generalized signs of infection (**Q2**).

The presence of a pelvic mass of the dimensions found is usually an indication for surgery. However, when the mass is caused by an abscess, there is a chance that it will respond to appropriate antibiotic therapy and resolve without the need for surgery. At the time of presentation, the decision as to whether to adopt a conservative approach will be determined by the general condition of the patient and, most particularly, whether there are signs of generalized peritonitis which may be life threatening. In the absence of such signs, a conservative approach is justified so long as you are very vigilant for signs of worsening illness (**Q3**).

C. *trachomatis* is currently the most important cause of acute pelvic inflammatory disease in the UK. It is associated with various complications, including Bartholin's abscess, eye problems and Reiter's disease. Fitz-Hugh–Curtis syndrome is perihepatitis with 'violin string' adhesions between the surface of the liver and the anterior abdominal wall (discussed further in case 36). It may be caused by *N. gonorrhoeae* as well as *C. trachomatis* (Wang *et al*, 1980). Chlamydial infection is not associated with peripheral neuropathy or Still's disease, the latter being rheumatoid arthritis in childhood in which splenomegaly, lymphadenopathy and pericarditis may occur (**Q4: true = A, B, C; false = D, E**).

Failure of the clinical signs to improve over 48 hours, particularly when there is no objective reduction in the size of the abscess on ultrasonography, is an indication for surgical intervention. Laparoscopic drainage would probably be unsuccessful, as it is important to break down all the loculi within the abscess cavity and not leave any pockets of pus behind. You should be as conservative as possible in a young woman with regard to removal of structures, and indeed oöphorectomy and hysterectomy in this situation may be extremely difficult (**Q5**).

With the development of chronic pelvic inflammatory disease associated with debilitating pain, the options for management are very limited in a 21 year old. Pelvic clearance has major implications both from the point of view of reproduction, even though her chances of spontaneous conception are extremely small, and also with regard to her menopausal status. The advice of a pain specialist would certainly be appropriate, but an attempt at adhesiolysis and particularly freeing the uterus in view of her dyspareunia may be worthwhile. There is no evidence that hormonal treatment has any role to play in this condition (**Q6: true = B, C; false = A, D**).

Ultimately, the only therapeutic option may be definitive surgery, which should involve total abdominal hysterectomy and bilateral salpingo-oöphorectomy, but clearly you should have explored all the other options in such a young woman before deciding on this. Such treatment is generally very effective in relieving symptoms. The woman should be counselled regarding hormone replacement therapy and it may be appropriate to offer egg retrieval and storage before surgery. A temptation to conserve an ovary should be resisted, as this would almost certainly need to be removed because of persistent pain within a relatively short time after the hysterectomy (**Q7**).

REFERENCE

Wang SP, Eschienbach DN, Holmes KK, Wager G, Grayston JF. *Chlamydia trachomatis* infection in Fitz-Hugh–Curtis syndrome. *Am J Obstet Gynecol* 1980; **138**: 1034–1038.

FACTS YOU SHOULD HAVE LEARNT . . .

▶ The presentation and management of acute pelvic inflammatory disease
▶ Complications of *Chlamydia trachomatis* infection
▶ The management of chronic pelvic inflammatory disease

CASE 38

An abnormal cervical smear

A 33-year-old P2 + 0 Caucasian woman attended her general practitioner's surgery for a routine cervical smear. A previous smear had been taken 3 years before and was reported as negative. She had no gynaecological symptoms and regular periods. She had had two children and used a coil for contraception. Examination was normal and the coil threads were present. The smear report read 'An inflammatory smear with *Actinomyces*-like organisms'. The general practitioner arranged to see the patient.

QI: Which of the following would have been appropriate action by the general practitioner?
A: Referral for colposcopy.
B: Antibiotics.
C: Removal of the coil.
D: Cryocautery to the cervix

After appropriate treatment, a further smear was taken 3 months later. This was reported as 'mild dyskaryosis'. The woman was extremely anxious when she was informed of the result.

Q2: How would you have counselled her?

She remained asymptomatic and reattended 6 months later for a further smear. She reported that she and her husband had not been very good at using sheaths and that her period was 2 weeks late. A pregnancy test was positive. Although the pregnancy was not planned, she decided to continue with it. The general practitioner repeated the smear, which was again reported as 'mild dyskaryosis'.

Q3: Which of the following would have been appropriate action by the general practitioner?
A: Repeat smear after the pregnancy.
B: Termination of the pregnancy.
C: Referral for colposcopy.

The patient experienced some postcoital bleeding on several occasions during the first trimester of pregnancy. She remained well otherwise and an ultrasound scan at 8 weeks of pregnancy confirmed an ongoing intrauterine gestation appropriate for her gestational age.

She attended the colposcopy clinic when she was 15 weeks' pregnant. The cervix appeared normal macroscopically, but following application of acetic acid the findings were described as acetowhite epithelium grade 2 with areas of mosaicism and punctation, and the squamocolumnar junction was visible.

Q4: Which of the following would have been optimal management?
A: Review in 4 months.
B: Review 2 months after delivery.
C: Punch biopsy of the abnormal epithelium.
D: Cone biopsy.

The pregnancy progressed well although the patient continued to have some postcoital bleeding. The placenta was found to be fundal on ultrasonographic imaging. Colposcopic assessment was unchanged at 32 weeks and a further appointment was made for 2 months after delivery. On this occasion, the acetowhite epithelium was described as grade 3 but the assessment was otherwise unchanged.

Q5: What should have been your management plan?
A: Review in 6 months.
B: Punch biopsy of the abnormal epithelium.
C: Large loop excision of the transformation zone (LLETZ).
D: Admission for staging of the disease.

The findings were discussed with the patient who considered that the problem had been going on for so long that she wished to have it sorted out as soon as possible. LLETZ was performed in the clinic under local anaesthetic. The procedure was uncomplicated and arrangements were made for a follow-up attendance at the colposcopy clinic six months later. The histology report on the specimen showed extensive cervical intraepithelial neoplasia (CIN) III with glandular involvement. There was no evidence of invasive carcinoma, but the abnormal epithelium extended to the ectocervical margin of excision whilst there was normal columnar epithelium at the endocervical excision margin.

Q6: What should have been your management plan?
A: Hysterectomy.
B: Knife cone biopsy.
C: Repeat colposcopy and cytology in 6 months.

The histology findings and its implications were discussed with the woman. She elected to be as conservative as possible. The colposcopic assessment was carried out 6 months later. There was a small area of acetowhite epithelium adjacent to the external cervical os, and columnar epithelium was visible above this. A biopsy confirmed CIN III and a smear was reported as 'severe dyskaryosis'.

Q7: What are the different management options?

An abdominal hysterectomy was performed. It was a straightforward procedure and the patient made a good recovery. The histology report showed a small area of CIN III at the external os, and the vaginal margins of the specimen revealed normal squamous epithelium.

Q8: What follow-up arrangements should you make?
A: No further smears are necessary.
B: Vault smears annually for 5 years.
C: Vault smears annually for life.
D: Vault smears at 6 and 18 months, and if negative no more.

COMMENTARY

Minor smear abnormalities do not require immediate referral for specialist investigation. Generally at least two, and probably three, smears showing abnormalities less severe than dyskaryosis should be performed before colposcopy is recommended. Inflammatory smears may be caused by infection, and swabs should be taken with appropriate antibiotic therapy, if indicated, before repeating the smear. In this case, *Actinomyces*-like organisms were detected. These are almost exclusively associated with the use of an intrauterine contraceptive device. The coil should have been removed and the smear repeated 3 months later. Had the second smear been normal, it would have been possible to reinsert the coil (**Q1: true = C; false = A, B, D**).

The second smear showed 'mild dyskaryosis' and the patient was understandably anxious. It is currently recommended that smears showing mild dyskaryosis should be repeated 6 months later (Duncan, 1992). There is, however, controversy regarding this because of the occurrence of high-grade CIN in many such cases and the concern that there is a significant risk of women defaulting from follow-up (Flanelly *et al*, 1994). The arguments against immediate referral include the risk of unnecessary interventions and increased anxiety for the woman. In counselling her, you should have been reassuring about the risks of serious disease and you should stress the fact that so long as she reattended there was no significant danger associated with adopting a conservative approach (**Q2**).

When the third smear showed 'mild dyskaryosis' again, the patient should have been referred for colposcopic assessment. Her pregnancy was not a contraindication to this. During pregnancy it is important to assess the cervix in order to exclude invasive carcinoma (**Q3: true = C; false = A, B**). Satisfactory colposcopy with visualization of the squamocolumnar junction is almost always possible in pregnancy as the columnar epithelium becomes more prominent on the visible part of the cervix. One does not treat CIN during pregnancy or indeed biopsy the cervix because of the increased vascularity unless there is suspicion of invasive carcinoma. In this situation, a wedge biopsy would usually be performed under general anaesthesia. Most colposcopists recommend continued surveillance during pregnancy because of concern about progression, although others argue that unless the colposcopic appearances are alarming the risk of progression to invasive disease is so small that further assessment can be deferred until after the pregnancy (**Q4: true = A, B; false = C, D**).

Following pregnancy and the puerperium, treatment can be carried out. In this case, a satisfactory colposcopy was performed with assessment of the whole transformation zone. The colposcopic diagnosis was CIN without suspicion of invasion. Either a punch biopsy before treatment or LLETZ would have been appropriate. The performance of LLETZ would have represented a 'see and treat' policy with the risk of unnecessary treatment particularly with less severe abnormalities. A punch biopsy would have confirmed that treatment was necessary. In view of the colposcopic impression of CIN III and the patient's anxiety, immediate treatment was reasonable (**Q5: true = B, C; false = A, D**).

With the diagnosis of CIN III extending to one of the excision margins, all three management options were acceptable. In this situation, the patient's views after counselling are very important. In the absence of invasive disease, the authors would favour option C. The chances of adequate treatment having been performed with such a histology report are approximately 70%. Even if residual CIN were present, the chances of it progressing to invasive disease during the following 6 months would be extremely small (**Q6: true = A, B, C**).

Six months later, when residual CIN was confirmed, excisional treatment was essential to ensure that all the abnormal epithelium had been removed. You cannot be confident of a satisfactory colposcopy after treatment as islands of squamous epithelium may be isolated above columnar epithelium during healing. The options for management would be LLETZ, knife cone biopsy or hysterectomy, and the patient's views should be considered during counselling. So long as adequate excision is achieved, the prognosis is excellent (**Q7**).

Following hysterectomy, vault smears should be performed at 6 and 18 months. It is not considered cost-effective to continue screening after this (**Q8: true = D; false = A, B, C**).

If the patient does have an abnormal smear following hysterectomy, the management is complicated. Colposcopic assessment of the vault should be performed with appropriate biopsies. If the biopsies confirm vaginal intraepithelial neoplasia (VAIN) the options are either conservative management, usually reserved for low-grade VAIN, or definitive treatment. In the past, laser ablation was advocated but this has been found to be inappropriate because of the risk of leaving VAIN above the vault suture line with the subsequent development of invasive cancer. The options are therefore surgical excision, more safely performed via an abdominal approach involving an extensive dissection of the bladder and ureters, or localized radiotherapy directed to the vagina. The former is preferred in younger patients with disease confined to the upper vagina, whereas the latter is favoured in other cases.

REFERENCES

Duncan ID. *NHS Screening Programme Guidelines for Clinic Practice and Programme Management.* Oxford: National Co-ordinating Network, 1992.

Flanelly G, Anderson D, Kitchener HC *et al.* Management of women with mild and moderate cervical dyskaryosis. *BMJ* 1994; **308**: 1399–1403.

FACTS YOU SHOULD HAVE LEARNT . . .

▶ **The management of minor smear abnormalities**
▶ **The management of actinomycosis diagnosed on cervical cytology**
▶ **The management of abnormal smears in pregnancy**
▶ **Options for treatment of CIN, both initial and recurrent disease**

CASE 39

Cervical cancer

A 39-year-old woman presented to her general practitioner with a 3-month history of an offensive, watery, blood-stained discharge and vaginal bleeding every day of varying amounts. Her cycles had been regular with no abnormal bleeding before this and she had had a negative cervical smear 2 years earlier. On examination she was overweight and there were no abdominal abnormalities. On passing a speculum, her general practitioner noted a large fungating tumour arising from the cervix which bled on contact. He arranged an urgent outpatient appointment at which the findings were confirmed.

QI: How would you counsel the patient?

She was admitted 1 week later and underwent a staging procedure.

Q2: Which of the following should be part of the staging procedure?
A: Cystoscopy.
B: Laparoscopy.
C: Proctoscopy.
D: Chest radiography.
E: Cervical biopsy.

Following the procedure, the stage of disease was IB. The histology of the tumour was a poorly differentiated squamous cell carcinoma with considerable vascular channel involvement.

Q3: Which of the following would be appropriate treatment options?
A: Radical pelvic radiotherapy.
B: Pelvic and whole abdominal radiotherapy.
C: Chemotherapy followed by radical surgery.
D: Total abdominal hysterectomy.
E: Wertheim's hysterectomy.

Q4: Which option would you have chosen and why?

Two weeks later, the patient was readmitted for a radical hysterectomy and pelvic lymphadenectomy (Wertheim's hysterectomy). A lower midline incision was performed. She had a narrow pelvis which combined with her obesity to make access to the pelvis difficult. There were no suspiciously enlarged lymph nodes and good macroscopic clearance of the tumour was achieved. She required a 4-unit blood transfusion. At the end of the procedure, a suprapubic catheter was inserted into the bladder and each side of the pelvis was drained with a Redivac suction tube.

Q5: What are the purposes of suprapubic catheterization and the pelvic drains?

In the week following surgery, the patient developed a fluctuating temperature with general malaise and lower abdominal pain. She felt bloated and had a poor appetite. Cultures from the wound, vagina, urine and sputum did not grow any significant organisms. Seven days after operation the wound became increasingly tender and, in spite of nylon being used to close the rectus sheath, the lower half of the wound dehisced completely.

She was taken back to theatre. The wound was fully opened, the remaining sutures were removed and a mass closure using nylon deep tension sutures was performed. In addition, interrupted nylon sutures were inserted into the sheath.

Whilst in theatre, the sheets were noted to be soaked by clear fluid. Vaginal assessment before reversing the anaesthetic did not reveal any obvious vaginal fistula, although clearly this was a major concern.

Q6: What would be your management following this procedure?

The patient gradually recovered and the wound inflammation resolved. The sutures were removed 10 days later with no further problem. Unfortunately, although the catheter was left on free drainage, there was increasing vaginal leakage. An intravenous pyelogram confirmed a vesicovaginal fistula.

Q7: How would you deal with this complication?

The histology report on the hysterectomy specimen confirmed a poorly differentiated squamous carcinoma with significant vascular channel involvement. The vaginal margins were more than 2 cm clear of the tumour, which did not extend into the parametrium or the body of the uterus. The lymph glands were all free of tumour.

Q8: Which of the following would you recommend?
A: Pelvic radiotherapy.
B: Platinum-based chemotherapy.
C: Combination of radiotherapy and chemotherapy.
D: No further treatment.

The vesicovaginal fistula was repaired successfully and 3 months later the woman was continent at all times.

Q9: How would you follow the patient up?

COMMENTARY

Whilst it is decreasing in incidence as a result of the effectiveness of the cervical screening programme, cervical cancer is the most important cause of abnormal vaginal bleeding in women under the age of 40 years. This patient presented with the classical symptoms of cervical cancer, namely prolonged vaginal bleeding and blood-stained watery discharge. The majority of young women with such symptoms will have dysfunctional bleeding, but this case demonstrates the importance of visualizing the cervix. A suspicious appearance is an indication for urgent referral. Cervical cytology may be unhelpful in this situation, as the inflammatory changes in the cervix as well as the blood-staining may mask the neoplastic cells.

Following the initial outpatient attendance, it is most important to counsel the woman appropriately as she needs to establish a trusting relationship with you at a very anxious time. You should make her aware of the likely diagnosis, the way in which this will be confirmed and the possible management. It is also essential that she knows that effective treatment is available and that, although she has a serious disease, there is a reasonable chance of cure (**Q1**).

The stage of disease is the most important prognostic factor and it is a matter of urgency that this be ascertained as soon as possible. Staging involves an examination under anaesthetic with vaginal and rectal assessment of tumour extension, cystoscopy, proctoscopy, biopsy of the tumour and intravenous pyelography (**Q2: true = A, C, E; false = B, D**).

This woman had a stage IB tumour – a clinically obvious lesion confined to the cervix. The usual treatment options are either radical pelvic radiotherapy or Wertheim's hysterectomy (**Q3: true = A, E; false = B, C, D**). There has not been a randomized trial comparing these treatment options, but the survival figures for each modality are similar in most series. The choice of treatment must therefore take into account the morbidity involved. The advantages of surgery are that the ovaries can be conserved, which is clearly important in younger women, and there is less sexual dysfunction compared with radiotherapy (Abitbol and Davenport, 1974). Radiotherapy causes transient bladder and bowel dysfunction, which rarely results in long-term problems, whereas surgery can cause long-term bladder dysfunction as well as the risk of fistula formation. Older patients may have medical problems that increase the risks of major surgery. On balance, you should generally favour surgical treatment in premenopausal women and radiotherapy in postmenopausal women. The main proviso with regard to surgical treatment is the risk of lymph node metastases. It is generally recommended that patients with positive lymph nodes should undergo postoperative radiotherapy as surgical lymphadenopathy is rarely complete (Kjorstad and Bond, 1984). Clearly, the morbidity of surgery followed by radiotherapy is considerably increased, and if you could accurately predict lymph node metastases then you should favour radical radiotherapy rather than surgery in such patients. Lymphangiography, magnetic resonance imaging, computed tomography (CT) and even fine-needle aspiration of nodes based on CT findings are not particularly accurate in diagnosing nodal metastases. Prognostic indicators for metastatic disease and survival include grade of disease, vascular channel involvement and large volume disease, and these may be useful in treatment planning (**Q4**).

If you embark on primary surgery, you should try to minimize complications by the appropriate use of prophylactic antibiotics and anticoagulants. Voiding problems are frequently encountered after surgery and the value of suprapubic bladder drainage is the avoidance of recurrent urethral catheterization with an increased risk of infection. In dissecting out the pelvic lymph nodes, the lymphatic drainage from the lower limbs is interrupted and large volumes of lymph accumulate in the pelvis. If the pelvis is not drained, there is a significant risk of lymphocyst formation, which may necessitate further surgery. Alternative lymphatic drainage from the legs is usually achieved within 1 week of surgery and the drains rarely have to be kept in longer than this (**Q5**).

Further surgical complications include fistula formation from the ureters or bladder. These usually result from avascular necrosis and infection, although they may be caused by surgical trauma. If you suspect vaginal leakage of urine, it is important to confirm this and to ascertain the cause, both for the patient's comfort and for the avoidance of long-term renal damage. Intravenous pyelography with cystoscopy is usually diagnostic, and the help of an experienced urological surgeon is essential (**Q6**). The first attempt at fistula repair is the one most likely to succeed. The optimum time is after 2 months when inflammation around the fistula site has settled and the tract has epithelialized (**Q7**).

The need for adjuvant treatment following surgery will be determined by the pathologist's findings. It is important to minimize the risks of both local and distant recurrence. If there is wide local clearance of tumour on the extended hysterectomy specimen and the lymph nodes are clear of tumour, then there is no advantage in giving any further treatment (**Q8: true = D; false = A, B, C**). The role of chemotherapy in cervical cancer remains to be defined.

Follow-up after initial treatment remains mainly clinical, as imaging techniques are of limited value. Vaginal vault smears are helpful in patients who have not undergone radiotherapy, but are difficult to interpret after radiotherapy. Patients should be reviewed every 3–6 months for 5 years, but there is only limited value in further follow-up (**Q9**).

REFERENCES

Abitbol MM, Davenport JH. Sexual dysfunction after therapy for cervical carcinoma. *Am J Obstet Gynecol* 1974; **119**: 181–189.

Kjorstad KE, Bond B. Stage IB adenocarcinoma of the cervix. *Am J Obstet Gynecol* 1984; **150**: 297–299.

FACTS YOU SHOULD HAVE LEARNT . . .

▶ The presentation and staging of cervical carcinoma
▶ The treatment options in cervical cancer and their indications
▶ The complications of treatment for this disease

CASE 40

Hormonal contraception

A 32-year-old woman presented to her general practitioner having recently undergone a termination of pregnancy following a 'sheath failure'. She had two children, aged 5 and 3 years, and was uncertain of what to do for contraception. In the past she had used an intrauterine contraceptive device, but this had been removed because of heavy irregular vaginal bleeding. She thought she would like the contraceptive pill but was concerned because of recent publicity regarding the increased risk of thrombosis.

Q1: What would you advise her regarding the risk of thrombosis?

Q2: Which of the following factors would adversely influence your prescribing the pill?
A: Current medication with sodium valproate.
B: Fibroids.
C: A family history of ovarian cancer.
D: Hepatitis B carrier status.
E: Past history of hypertension in pregnancy.

There were no contraindications in her history to prescribing the combined pill. On examination, she weighed 60 kg and the blood pressure was 110/70 mmHg. The doctor gave her 3 months' supply of the combined contraceptive pill Ovranette (ethinyloestradiol 30 µg, levonorgestrel 150 µg) and arranged to review her after this time. She had found it difficult to remember to take the pill every day and consequently had experienced several episodes of breakthrough bleeding. In addition, she complained of dryness of her skin with mild acne as well as loss of libido.

Q3: Which of the following are progestogenic side-effects of the combined pill?
A: Vaginal dryness.
B: Breast tenderness.
C: Loss of libido.
D: Increased vaginal discharge.
E: Headaches.

The patient did not consider that she could continue using Ovranette because of the side-effects, but she was keen to carry on with hormonal contraception.

Q4: Would you advise a different combined pill or suggest changing to the progestogen-only pill?

After thorough counselling regarding the options, she opted to take the combined preparation Femodene (ethinyloestradiol 30 μg, gestodene 75 μg). Six weeks later, her general practitioner was called out to see her with an episode of gastroenteritis. She had experienced diarrhoea and vomiting for 48 hours. The general practitioner prescribed a rehydrating agent and withdrawal of solid food until the symptoms had settled.

Q5: What advice would you have given regarding contraception?

After taking Femodene for 3 months, her compliance had improved but she was still missing one or two pills each month. She was desperate to avoid pregnancy and said she would like to be more secure than at present.

Q6: What are the available options?

The patient did not want anything as permanent as sterilization, even though she had recently undergone a termination of pregnancy and did not currently anticipate wishing to have any more children. Although she had discontinued using the coil in the past, she thought she would like to try a Mirena intrauterine delivery system (with levonorgestrel).

Q7: What are the advantages and disadvantages of the Mirena coil?

Three months later, she complained of persistent spotting of blood on most days. She had had a normal period after the first month, but could not identify a period since that time.

Q8: How would you counsel her?

The patient agreed to continue with the Mirena coil and 6 months later she had not had any bleeding at all for 3 months. She was worried about becoming pregnant but was reassured by the reported efficacy of this form as contraception as well as the fact that amenorrhoea is a common occurrence.

Q9: How else may progestogens be given?

COMMENTARY

There is an increased risk of thrombosis with any use of the pill. However, there are specific factors that increase the risks considerably and these include obesity, varicose veins, previous history of thrombosis and smoking. In addition, it has been shown that the progestogens, gestodene and desogestrel, add a twofold increase in the risk of venous thrombosis compared with the combined pill containing other progestogens. Ovranette contains levonorgestrel (**Q1**).

Certain drugs, particularly those used in the treatment of epilepsy, cause enzyme induction, and higher doses of oestrogen are required to achieve adequate contraception. However, sodium valproate is not an enzyme-inducing drug. The combined pill has no adverse effect on fibroids and has been found to protect against ovarian cancer. Abnormal liver function may be a contraindication to use of the pill, but being a hepatitis B carrier is not in itself an adverse factor. Patients with a history of hypertensive disease in pregnancy are at increased risk of subsequent development of essential hypertension, and blood pressure should be monitored closely in such patients wishing to take the combined oral contraceptive pill (**Q2: true = E; false = A, B, C, D**).

Side-effects of the contraceptive pill may be related to either the progestogen or the oestrogen component. The former may cause vaginal dryness, acne, amenorrhoea and loss of libido, whilst the latter may result in fluid retention, breast tenderness, vaginal discharge and headaches (**Q3: true = A, C; false = B, D, E**).

If a woman has a problem with compliance on the combined pill then you should be reluctant for her to use the progestogen-only pill. This relies on much greater patient control for effectiveness and should be taken at the same time each day. The problems this woman encountered were related to progestogenic side-effects and these may be more marked if she goes on to the progestogen-only pill. Combined pills containing gestodene and desogestrel tend to result in less marked progestogen-related problems, and in a patient without increased risk factors for venous thrombosis gestodene-containing preparations may be appropriate (**Q4**).

When a woman forgets to take her pills, or has sickness which may result in failure of absorption, she requires additional precautions and one would employ the '7-day rule', using additional methods (probably sheaths) for 7 days after the last forgotten pill or the end of the sickness (**Q5**).

In a case of lack of compliance with contraceptive usage, barrier methods and pills are best avoided. Sterilization may be an option if the individual has no wish for further pregnancies but appropriate counselling is of the utmost importance. Intrauterine contraceptive devices are a possibility, but this patient had had one removed in the past because of bleeding problems. The new Mirena (intrauterine delivery system with levonorgestrel) may be an option. Other possible types of contraception would be progestogen-only contraceptives such as injections of Depo-Provera or a progestogen implant (Norplant) (**Q6**).

The Mirena coil is an intrauterine delivery system that combines the foreign body mechanism of action with that of hormonal contraception. It releases about 20 µg of levonorgestrel into the uterus each day and is licensed currently for 3 years. Its main advantages over a traditional intrauterine contraceptive device are decreased menstrual blood loss and a low risk of ectopic pregnancy and pelvic inflammatory disease. The main disadvantages are its initial cost of about £100 and initial spotting for up to 90 days, which may decrease compliance and hence the overall cost of contraception (**Q7**). It is important to warn patients about initial spotting and to reassure them that it will usually settle down and may result in prolonged amenorrhoea (**Q8**).

Other methods of giving progestogens include injections of Depo-Provera given 3 monthly, and the use of a progestogen implant. Both methods are very effective and useful in non-compliant women. Both may cause irregular bleeding, which is usually not heavy, and there may be subsequent amenorrhoea. Norplant is licensed for 5 years and is said to be almost 100% effective for the first 2 years and 98% effective for the whole 5-year period. It consists of five Silastic capsules inserted intradermally, most commonly in the upper arm. In addition to progestogenic side-effects, local skin reactions may occur and occasionally there may be chronic pain at the site of insertion. Removal may be difficult and individuals should receive specific training in this technique (**Q9**).

FACTS YOU SHOULD HAVE LEARNT . . .

▶ **Complications and side-effects of the combined oral contraceptive pill**
▶ **A rational approach to the use of hormonal contraception**
▶ **The different types of progestogen-only contraception**
▶ **The advantages and disadvantages of the levonorgestrel intrauterine delivery system (Mirena)**

CASE 41

Ovarian cyst

A 25-year-old P0+0 woman was admitted as an emergency with a 6-hour history of severe pain in the right iliac fossa. She had had similar episodes of pain during the preceding month but they had never lasted longer than 20 minutes at a time. She felt sick although she had no other gastrointestinal symptoms. Her last menstrual period had started 3 weeks earlier and had been normal. She took the progestogen-only pill for contraception.

On examination, she had a tachycardia of 120 beats per minute (bpm) but she was normotensive (110/70 mmHg). Her temperature was 37.2°C. On abdominal palpation she was very tender with guarding in the right iliac fossa but the abdomen was otherwise soft. There were no abdominal masses palpable. On vaginal and rectal examination she was very tender on the right side and there was a suggestion of a right-sided swelling.

> **Q1:   Which of the following should be included in the differential diagnosis?**
> A: Appendicitis.
> B: Cholecystitis.
> C: Ectopic pregnancy.
> D: Complicated ovarian cyst.
> E: Pyelonephritis.

> **Q2:   What investigations would you perform?**

The patient required pethidine to control the pain. The haemoglobin level was 12.5 g dl^{-1} and the white cell count was 7×10^9 l^{-1}. Urine testing was negative, as was a human chorionic gonadotrophin assay. An ultrasound scan showed a 5 × 6-cm unilocular cystic swelling in the right fornix apparently arising from the ovary. The uterus was normal in size and the other ovary appeared normal.

> **Q3:   What are the possible complications that could have occurred to the cyst and which do you think is most likely?**

> **Q4:   How would you counsel the patient?**

Arrangements were made to take the patient to theatre for a laparoscopy. Depending on the laparoscopic findings she would either have the cyst removed laparoscopically, or via a laparotomy.

An uncomplicated laparoscopy was performed at which the right ovarian cyst was confirmed. The ovary and tube had undergone torsion and both were gangrenous. The left adnexa was normal.

Q5:   How would you proceed?

Two further incisions were made, the first in the right iliac fossa and the second in the midline suprapubically. Trocars were inserted through both incisions and the tube and ovary were picked up in grasping forceps via the midline trocar. A catgut loop was passed through the right-sided trocar and this was fed around the tube and ovary after the cyst was decompressed using a spinal needle and syringe. The tube and ovary were grasped again with the forceps passing through the loop, and the latter was tightened around the base of the tube and ovary, incorporating all the gangrenous tissue. The catgut loop was then cut with scissors. Another loop was applied in the same way. The tube and ovary were cut off above the loops whilst being grasped firmly. A pincer instrument was passed through the midline incision outside the trocar and the latter was removed with the grasping forceps holding the tube and ovary whilst stretching the incision. The tube and ovary were sent for histological assessment. The pelvis was irrigated with warm saline and the pedicle was inspected carefully to ensure haemostasis before removing the laparoscope. The incisions were closed with polyglactin.

Q6:   What are the potential early complications relating to laparoscopic salpingo-oöphorectomy?

The patient was observed overnight and felt much better the following day. She was allowed home and returned for review 6 weeks later.

When she was reviewed at the follow-up visit, she was asymptomatic and findings on examination were unremarkable. However, she was very concerned about her fertility.

Q7:   How would you counsel her?

She was discharged from the clinic, but returned 3 months later complaining of intermittent colicky pain in the region of the incision in the right iliac fossa.

Q8:   What is the differential diagnosis?

Q9:   What further information do you require?

Findings on examination were unremarkable and the patient was advised to use simple analgesics as necessary. She was seen 3 months later when the episode of pain seemed to have settled. She was discharged from the clinic.

COMMENTARY

The symptoms and signs at initial presentation in this patient suggest some sort of pathological process occurring in the right iliac fossa or right fornix. They are not specific to any one system and the suggestion of a mass would favour a diagnosis of a complicated ovarian cyst or an appendix abscess. An ectopic pregnancy should also be considered although it is unusual to feel a mass on bimanual examination. Pyelonephritis is much less likely, and cholecystitis is extremely improbable (**Q1: true = A, C, D; false = B, E**).

Your investigations should be aimed at the above differential diagnosis, as well as a possible pelvic infection. They should include a full blood count, urine culture, vaginal and endocervical swabs, a pregnancy test and pelvic ultrasonography, preferably performed with a vaginal probe (**Q2**).

The finding of a cystic swelling of 5 × 6 cm confirms the cause of the problem. Possible emergency complications of an ovarian cyst are torsion, rupture, haemorrhage and infection. In this case rupture had clearly not occurred. Infection was unlikely in view of her temperature, which was almost normal. In addition, in the presence of an infected cyst, you might expect some signs on the left side. Haemorrhage or torsion are both possibilities, but the authors would favour the latter because of the history of previous episodes of similar short-lasting pain over the preceding few weeks. This suggests that the cyst was twisting and untwisting intermittently before finally undergoing complete torsion (**Q3**).

The fact that the cyst may have undergone torsion, and her need for opiate analgesics, meant that surgical intervention was necessary. You should discuss the need for surgery with the patient as well as the possible interventions. Torsion may have caused the ovary to become gangrenous, necessitating its removal. If this were not the case, you may be able to remove the cyst and conserve the ovary. You should also discuss the possibility of performing the whole procedure laparoscopically whilst making it clear that this may not be technically possible and a laparotomy may be required. The likelihood of such a unilocular cyst in a young woman being malignant is so remote that the authors would not even discuss pelvic clearance in this situation (**Q4**).

Having found a gangrenous tube and ovary at laparoscopy, you have no choice but to remove both organs, and the decision to be made is whether or not this can be achieved laparoscopically. Such a decision depends on the surgeon's ability and experience as well as on factors such as mobility of the adnexa. In this case there were no adhesions limiting mobility and the procedure was carried out laparoscopically using catgut endoloops fed over the tube and ovary and tied beneath them (**Q5**).

The operation was performed without complication and a careful inspection to ensure haemostasis was made before removing the instruments. The most likely early complication of laparoscopic salpingo-oöphorectomy would be haemorrhage from a slipped pedicle. The chances of this would be reduced by using two catgut endoloops around the base of the tube and ovary. Damage to bowel may present early, although this would be less likely in the absence of diathermy being used during the procedure. Ureteric damage would also be unlikely to present within the first 24 hours after surgery (**Q6**).

It is generally believed that ovarian function can be maintained satisfactorily with one ovary and the fact that the left adnexa was normal was reassuring. The main risk to fertility would be due to adhesions resulting in distortion of the remaining tube. The chances of this happening after an uncomplicated laparoscopic salpingo-oöphorectomy are small and you should be reassuring to the woman regarding her subsequent fertility. A slight concern would be the occurrence of a torted cyst on the other side. The authors are not aware of any publications relating to this and have not come across this problem in their practices. You should, however, warn the patient to present early if she ever developed similar pain on the left side (**Q7**).

A late complication of laparoscopic surgery is the development of hernia through the small trocar incisions. It is important to suture the muscle sheath incisions in the wounds at the time of surgery. You should also be concerned about possible bowel obstruction (**Q8**). You should thus enquire about the presence of any bowel symptoms such as distension and vomiting. In the absence of any such symptoms and a failure to demonstrate an incisional hernia, you should be reassuring to the patient in this situation. Fortunately, her symptoms settled spontaneously and she had no further problems (**Q9**).

FACTS YOU SHOULD HAVE LEARNT . . .

- ▶ **The diffential diagnosis of right iliac fossa pain**
- ▶ **The complications of ovarian cysts**
- ▶ **The advantages and disadvantages of laparoscopic oöphorectomy**

CASE 42

Pelvic mass

A 47-year-old woman presented to her general practitioner with a 6-month history of increasing abdominal swelling with tightness of her clothing. He found a smooth rounded mass arising from the pelvis and extending to the umbilicus. There was no abdominal tenderness and no other palpable mass. There was no lymphadenopathy.

The patient was referred urgently for a gynaecological opinion. She had no specific symptoms, in particular: her menstrual periods were regular with no abnormal bleeding; she had had a negative smear within the last year. The abdominal findings were confirmed and vaginal examination revealed a smooth swelling anterior to the rectum with the cervix pushed forwards and the uterus difficult to define.

Q1:   What is the differential diagnosis?

Q2:   Which of the following investigations should you perform?
      A: Computed tomography (CT) of the abdomen and pelvis.
      B: Ultrasound scan of the abdomen and pelvis.
      C: Pelvic lymphangiography.
      D: Serum CA125 assay.
      E: Lupus anticoagulant.

Following investigation, the diagnosis of a left ovarian cyst was made.

Q3:   Which of the following features would be suggestive of malignancy.
      A: Solid areas within the cyst.
      B: Teeth within the cyst.
      C: Free peritoneal fluid.
      D: A loaded large bowel.
      E: A CA125 level of 175 IU l^{-1}.

The cyst contained solid areas, there was a small amount of free fluid in the pouch of Douglas and the CA125 level was 175 IU l^{-1}. The cyst did not contain any teeth and the bowel was loaded with faeces.

Q4:   How would you counsel this patient?

Q5:   Which of the following would you recommend before surgery?
      A: Chest radiography.
      B: Liver function tests.
      C: A clotting screen.
      D: Bowel preparation.

Q6: What is the aim of surgery in this case?

At operation, there was a small amount of ascitic fluid which was sampled and sent for cytological assessment. A smooth-surfaced mobile tumour, approximately 20 cm in diameter, arising from the left ovary was removed along with a normal-looking ovary and the uterus. In addition, an infracolic omentectomy was performed. There was no evidence of any disease apart from the ovarian tumour.

The patient made a good recovery, and the pathology report revealed: 'A 20-cm diameter tumour arising from the left ovary containing a mucinous cystadenocarcinoma, moderately differentiated, with tumour just breaking the capsule in one area. The right ovary and uterus were microscopically normal. The omentum contained several microscopic deposits of adenocarcinoma cells identical to those in the left ovary.'

The cytology report of the ascitic fluid revealed several clumps of adenocarcinoma cells.

Q7: What is the stage of disease, and how would you manage the patient now?

Following chemotherapy, arrangements were made to review the patient every 3 months for 2 years and subsequently to reduce the frequency of attendance until she was discharged after 5 years.

Q8: At each follow-up visit, which of the following investigations should you carry out?
A: Perform a clotting screen.
B: Arrange a CT scan.
C: Take serum for CA125 assay.
D: Perform chest radiography.

COMMENTARY

The two most likely diagnoses in this case would be an ovarian tumour or a large fibroid uterus. However, in a premenopausal woman you must always remember that she could be pregnant. You may occasionally be caught out by a chronically distended bladder due to urinary retention. Other pelvic masses include bladder tumours, pelvic kidneys and gastrointestinal tumours, although these rarely present in this way and tend not to be smoothly enlarged (**Q1**).

The most useful investigation would be an ultrasound scan of the abdomen and pelvis, possibly combined with colour Doppler imaging (Bourne *et al*, 1989). It would have confirmed the diagnosis in this case. Following this, serum should have been taken for CA125 assay, whilst measurement of lupus anticoagulant would not have been relevant. A CT scan and pelvic lymphangiography may have given additional information but the authors would not have recommended these expensive investigations as the information they provide would have been obtained at subsequent laparotomy (**Q2: true = B, D; false = A, C, E**).

Features suggestive of malignancy would have been solid areas within the cyst, free peritoneal fluid and a CA125 level greater than 65 IU l^{-1}. However, none of these would have been conclusive evidence of malignancy. Whilst no marker is completely specific for epithelial ovarian cancer, CA125 is the most useful marker and is expressed by more than 80% of such tumours (Bast *et al*, 1983). It is important to take 10 ml of blood for CA125 estimation before surgery as the level may fall rapidly afterwards and the knowledge that a tumour expresses this marker is particularly useful in follow-up after treatment (**Q3: true = A, C, E; false = B, D**).

In counselling the patient it is important to emphasize that the cyst is arising from one of her ovaries. There is a possibility that it may be a cancer of the ovary, although you will know for certain only after the cyst has been removed and examined histologically. You must base your management on the assumption that it is cancer until this diagnosis has been categorically confirmed or refuted, as otherwise you risk treating the patient inappropriately. The correct treatment is to arrange a laparotomy as soon as possible, but certainly within 3–4 weeks. The operation involves a vertical incision in the lower abdomen with the aim of removing the uterus, both ovaries and some fatty tissue from the bowel, which is the commonest site of spread outside the pelvis. If there is any disease elsewhere, you should try to remove it all. If the cyst is malignant, she may need some chemotherapy. She will need to take hormone replacement therapy after the operation, regardless of the diagnosis (**Q4**).

Before operating, you should normally perform chest radiography, looking for evidence of a pleural effusion (Meig's syndrome), as well as liver function tests which may be altered by metastatic disease. Whilst blood coagulation may be altered in advanced malignant disease, you should not arrange a clotting screen unless the platelet count is grossly altered. Bowel preparation, usually with Klean-prep is important as it is difficult to predict bowel involvement and the likely need for a bowel movement. Should this be necessary, you are then in a position to perform a re-anastomosis rather than a defunctioning colostomy (**Q5: true = A, B, D; false = C**).

The purpose of the operation is to treat the condition and to carry out a staging procedure if the tumour is malignant. In ovarian cancer, the disease is staged surgically and therefore all patients should undergo a surgical procedure unless they are medically unfit to do so. The stage of disease is vitally important to know as this has implications not only for further management but also for prognosis (**Q6**).

In this case, the patient had stage III disease. Whilst macroscopic clearance of the tumour had been achieved, there may have been residual microscopic disease in the peritoneal cavity. Without further treatment, the risk of recurrence would be high and you should advise the patient to have adjuvant therapy. The options would be chemotherapy or whole abdominal radiotherapy. In the UK, chemotherapy is favoured, because it is believed to carry less morbidity for the patient. There is general agreement that six courses of platinum-based chemotherapy, usually carboplatin (dose: 400 mg ml^{-2}), over a 6-month period should be given, but there is less agreement about whether it should be given as a single agent or in combination with other drugs, usually an alkylating agent such as cyclophosphamide (dose: 750 mg ml^{-2}). Combination chemotherapy appears to confer a slight survival advantage, but this is at the cost of increased morbidity (**Q7**).

The overall 5-year survival rate for stage III disease is approximately 30%. However, this includes patients with macroscopic spread of tumour and such residual disease after surgery. In this patient's case, the chance of cure with adjuvant chemotherapy would probably approach 50%.

The purpose of follow-up is controversial. Apart from the disease itself, this patient would develop menopausal symptoms and should be given hormone replacement therapy in the form of unopposed oestrogen. There is no evidence that this has an adverse effect on the disease and there has been a suggestion that it may be beneficial (Eeler *et al*, 1992).

With regard to recurrence of cancer, the ability to detect clinical recurrence is poor and even sophisticated imaging techniques such as CT and magnetic resonance imaging are often unhelpful. One may use these if recurrence is suspected, but not routinely. The expression of CA125 may be of value, as this usually rises several months before recurrent disease becomes clinically apparent. Chest radiography may be used if clinically indicated, but clotting studies are not relevant (**Q8: true = C; false = A, B, D**).

The other problem with follow-up of patients with ovarian cancer after surgery and adjuvant chemotherapy is that further treatment options have been very limited until recently. However, the new drug paclitaxel (Taxol) does appear to offer useful second-line treatment in recurrent disease, and may also become the treatment of choice along with carboplatin in initial adjuvant therapy. Paclitaxel is currently very expensive and in any health-care system with limited resources will undoubtedly stimulate considerable debate as to its appropriate usage.

REFERENCES

Bast RC, Klug TC, St John E *et al*. A radioimmunoassay using a monoclonal antibody to monitor the course of epithelial ovarian cancer. *N Engl J Med* 1983; **309**: 833–837.

Bourne T, Campbell S, Steer C, Whitehead MI, Collins WP. Transvaginal colour flow imaging: a possible new screening technique for ovarian cancer. *BMJ* 1989; **299**: 1367–1370.

Eeler RA, Tam S, Fryatt I *et al*. Hormone replacement therapy and survival after surgery for ovarian cancer. *BMJ* 1992; **302**: 259–262.

FACTS YOU SHOULD HAVE LEARNT . . .

▶ The investigation and differential diagnosis of a pelvic mass
▶ The investigation, management and prognosis of epithelial ovarian cancer

CASE 43

Postmenopausal bleeding

A 54-year-old woman presented to her general practitioner after having been on tibolone for menopausal symptoms during the previous 2 years. Her periods had ceased at the age of 49 years and she had not bled again before starting hormone replacement therapy. She had experienced occasional vaginal spotting during the first 3 months on tibolone but was then free of any bleeding until 2 weeks before seeing her doctor. She had noted bleeding, with the blood loss similar to that of a period, for 5 days and had continued to have spotting for a further week. She had just stopped bleeding at the time of her consultation. A cervical smear taken 6 months earlier had been negative.

On examination, there were no abdominal abnormalities. The vagina was atrophic, the cervix looked healthy, the uterus was small and mobile, and there were no pelvic masses.

QI: What is the most likely cause of the bleeding?
   A: Endometrial cancer.
   B: Atrophic vaginitis.
   C: Tibolone hormone replacement therapy.
   D: Ovarian cancer.
   E: Endometrial polyp.

Q2:   What are the indications for using tibolone?

The general practitioner advised her to discontinue tibolone therapy. He arranged for her to have pelvic ultrasonography performed. This revealed a small uterus with endometrial thickness of 4 mm and normal ovaries.

Q3:   How would you manage the patient?

When she was seen in the general practitioner's surgery 2 months later there had been no further bleeding, but she was experiencing troublesome hot flushes. The doctor advised her to restart the tibolone treatment which was effective in alleviating the symptoms. Unfortunately she had further vaginal bleeding for 5 days 1 month later and she again reported this to the general practitioner. Examination findings were unchanged, but he advised her to discontinue the tibolone and arranged an urgent appointment with a consultant gynaecologist.

She was seen at the hospital 2 weeks later where the general practitioner's examination findings were confirmed.

Q4: Which of the following management plans would you advise?

A: Total abdominal hysterectomy and bilateral salpingo-oöphorectomy.

B: No further hormone replacement therapy and review in 3 months.

C: Diagnostic hysteroscopy and biopsy.

D: Prostaglandin therapy.

E: Combined hormone replacement therapy.

The patient was admitted 2 weeks later as a day case. A hysteroscopy was performed under general anaesthetic. This revealed a tumour approximately 2 cm in diameter on the anterior wall of the uterus, just above the internal cervical os. A biopsy was taken and sent for urgent examination. The report confirmed an adenocarcinoma that was moderately differentiated.

Q5: Which of the following would you recommend?

A: Total abdominal hysterectomy and bilateral salpingo-oöphorectomy.

B: Radical pelvic radiotherapy.

C: Wertheim's hysterectomy.

D: High-dose medroxyprogesterone acetate (Provera) followed 2 months later by pelvic clearance.

Arrangements were made to admit the patient for surgery 4 weeks later. At operation, the uterus was mobile with the serosal surface intact and the ovaries were normal in size and appearance. There were no palpable pelvic or para-aortic lymph nodes. The findings at laparotomy were normal. The uterus and ovaries were removed and she made a good recovery.

Histological examination confirmed a moderately differentiated adenocarcinoma. The tumour extended into the myometrium superficially and did not involve the cervix. There was a small focus of identical tumour in the right ovary.

The situation was explained to the woman, who agreed to undergo a course of pelvic radiotherapy.

Q6: What are the criteria for giving postoperative radiotherapy in patients with endometrial cancer?

The patient experienced quite severe diarrhoea during radiotherapy, and was managed with symptomatic treatment and rehydration. The diarrhoea resolved during the month after completion of the irradiation.

When reviewed 3 months after operation, the patient was well and was gradually resuming normal activities.

Q7: Which of the following management plans would you advise?

A: No further treatment.

B: Six cycles of carboplatin.

C: Medroxyprogesterone acetate.

D: Tamoxifen.

The patient was reviewed 3 months later. She had made an excellent recovery and the findings on examination were normal. She was, however, complaining of very troublesome hot sweats.

Q8:   How would you manage this problem?

COMMENTARY

The commonest cause of postmenopausal bleeding is atrophic vaginitis. However, in a woman of 54 who is taking hormone replacement therapy, the most likely cause is iatrogenic, due to the hormone preparation (**Q1: true = C; false = A, B, D, E**). Tibolone has oestrogenic, progestogenic and androgenic properties. Its role is in the management of vasomotor menopausal symptoms. It is not recommended for use until more than 12 months after the most recent period. The main advantage of tibolone therapy is the lack of a withdrawal bleed (**Q2**).

Historically, the only way of excluding endometrial malignancy was to curette the endometrium. However, with increasingly sophisticated ultrasound imaging techniques, it is now possible to exclude such a diagnosis by means of ultrasonographic assessment of endometrial thickness. A measurement of less than 6 mm is reassuring (Nasn *et al*, 1991). In this case the scan result was satisfactory and the authors would not have referred the patient at this stage (**Q3**). It would have been prudent to discontinue the tibolone for a few months, as no further bleeding after cessation of therapy would suggest that tibolone was indeed the cause of the problem. After 2 months, with the return of symptoms, reintroduction of the tibolone treatment was acceptable. When the patient bled again, specialist referral was appropriate. At this point, exploration of the uterine cavity would be essential (**Q4: true = C; false = A, B, D, E**).

The finding of a moderately differentiated adenocarcinoma on the anterior wall of the uterine body suggested a stage I lesion and the appropriate treatment was total abdominal hysterectomy and bilateral salpingo-oöphorectomy initially. There is no evidence that more radical surgery should be performed in stage I disease. Whilst the tumour is radiosensitive, survival is better when surgery is used rather than radical radiotherapy, and you should recommend the latter only in patients who are unfit for surgery. There is no evidence of benefit from high-dose progestogen therapy in stage I disease (**Q5: true = A; false = B, C, D**).

Following surgery and histological assessment of the specimen, the tumour was found to be stage III by virtue of the microscopic ovarian involvement. This was surprising, particularly as the primary tumour was not of high grade or penetrating deeply into the myometrium. The indications for postoperative pelvic radiotherapy are related to the risk of lymph node metastases. In stage II and III disease, such postoperative therapy would be recommended in most cases. In patients with stage IV disease, the treatment is dependent on the clinical findings and extent of disease. Pelvic nodes are involved by tumour in about 10% of clinical stage I disease overall (Buronow *et al*, 1984). The risk factors for nodal metastases include high-grade tumours and those invading deeply through the myometrium, and patients with stage I disease and these risk factors would be treated with adjuvant radiotherapy (**Q6**).

Over the past two decades, the use of high-dose progestogen therapy has been widely advocated in this disease. It would now appear that such treatment in early stage disease is inappropriate and that it should be reserved for patients with more advanced disease. In stage III disease you should advise this treatment for approximately 2 years after operation. Tamoxifen has also been shown to be of some benefit and this would be an alternative. Hormonal therapy appears to offer more benefit than cytotoxic chemotherapy in endometrial cancer (**Q7: true = C, D; false = A, B**).

The occurrence of hot sweats following treatment is not uncommon in perimenopausal women. Whilst endometrial cancer is a hormone-dependent tumour, there is no evidence that giving hormone replacement therapy increases the risk of recurrence. The authors would be cautious in their approach to this problem, but would give such treatment after appropriate counselling if the symptoms were troublesome. They would favour tibolone rather than unopposed oestrogen or combined oestrogen–progestogen preparations (**Q8**).

REFERENCES

Buronow RC, Morrow CP, Crossman WT *et al.* Surgical staging in endometrial cancer: clinical pathological findings of a prospective study. *Obstet Gynecol* 1984: **63**; 825–832.

Nasn MN, Shepherd JH, Setchell ME *et al.* The role of vaginal scan in measurement of endometrial thickness in postmenopausal women. *Br J Obstet Gynaecol* 1991; **98**; 470–475.

FACTS YOU SHOULD HAVE LEARNT . . .

▶ **The investigation of postmenopausal bleeding**
▶ **The management of endometrial carcinoma**

CASE 44

Hormone replacement therapy

A 50-year-old P3 + 0 Caucasian woman attended her general practitioner's surgery concerned that her mother had recently been admitted to hospital with a fractured femur at the age of 70 years. She had heard that old people developed weak bones that could be prevented by taking hormone replacement therapy (HRT) and she wanted to discuss this option.

QI: Which of the following are risk factors for developing osteoporosis?
A: Obesity.
B: Late menopause.
C: Polycystic ovarian syndrome.
D: Smoking.
E: Bed rest.

The patient had no particular risk factors for developing osteoporosis. Her menstrual cycles were still regular, and she weighed 65 kg with a height of 1.4 m. She did not complain of any menopausal symptoms.

Q2: How would you advise her?

She had some concerns about the risks of HRT and, although the doctor was reassuring about the association with breast cancer particularly when taken for less than 10 years. She was swayed by the fact that a close friend had recently been diagnosed with this condition. She decided that she would have a hormone test to see whether she was menopausal. The follicle stimulating hormone (FSH) level was 8 IU l^{-1}. After discussing these results with her general practitioner, she decided not to take HRT for the time being.

During the following 12 months, her cycles became increasingly irregular, varying between 21 and 35 days. In addition, her periods became heavier until she finally bled continuously for 3 weeks. At this stage she returned to see her general practitioner and requested that he prescribe her HRT.

Q3: How would you manage this problem?

She attended her local hospital and was seen by a consultant gynaecologist who arranged for an ultrasound scan of her pelvis to be carried out. This showed a normal-sized uterus with an endometrium of 8 mm in thickness. The ovaries were both normal with a small follicle in the right ovary. The gynaecologist performed an endometrial biopsy with a pipelle endometrial sampling device and arranged to review her a fortnight later.

The histology confirmed that the endometrium was proliferative with areas of simple cystic hyperplasia and no atypia.

Q4: Which of the following statements regarding simple cystic hyperplasia of the endometrium are correct?
A: It will progress to invasive cancer in 20% of cases if not treated.
B: Management should be by hysterectomy.
C: HRT is not contraindicated.
D: Active treatment may not be required.
E: A full curettage of the uterus should be performed.

The gynaecologist was concerned about giving HRT in this situation and decided that, as she was not having any menopausal symptoms, he would rather give her three cycles of progestogen therapy to try to regulate the bleeding pattern.

Three months later, she reported that the cycles had become regular and the periods were less heavy. The hormone treatment was therefore stopped and she was asked to return to the clinic in another 3 months.

At this time her menstrual cycles had remained normal with no intermenstrual bleeding. She requested that her menopausal status be checked again, and the FSH was level 20 IU l^{-1}. In view of this and the fact that her mother had recently fractured her wrist, she decided that she would like to take HRT. She was prescribed sequential preparations with 1 mg of oestradiol valerate for 16 days and 12 days of oestradiol valerate 1 mg and 75 µg of levonorgestrel and advised to see her general practitioner for further prescriptions. In his letter, the gynaecologist suggested that she should be referred back in the event of any more abnormal bleeding.

Unfortunately, the patient developed considerable abdominal bloating on the HRT and, after three cycles, she returned to her doctor for advice. She was not at all keen on remaining on the hormone tablets, but was equally concerned about her risk of osteoporosis.

Q5: How would you advise her?

She decided to have her bone mineral density assessment and would make a decision about whether to recommence HRT.

Q6: Which of the following techniques can be used to assess bone mineral density (BMD)?
A: Plain radiography.
B: Ultrasound scanning.
C: Magnetic resonance imaging.
D: Dual-photon absorptiometry.

Dual-photon absorptiometry was performed and this revealed normal levels of trabecular bone in the lumbar spine and cortical bone in the proximal femur.

She decided not to restart HRT, but over the subsequent few months she started to have increasingly troublesome night sweats and hot flushes. This prompted her to change her mind and she was commenced on Estracombi skin patches, which were effective. In addition, she tolerated this method of delivery much better than the oral preparation.

Q7:   Why do hot flushes and hot sweats occur?

This woman remained well over the next year with no symptoms and a regular withdrawal bleed. At a routine mammography examination, a 2 cm cyst was found in the right breast. This was aspirated and found to be benign. The patient was frightened by this and wondered whether there was an alternative to oestrogen therapy to alleviate her symptoms and help to prevent osteoporosis.

Q8:   How would you advise her?

She decided to take tibolone which was effective in controlling the night sweats. After 3 months without any bleeding, she had some spotting every day for 3 weeks. She was referred back to the hospital where a pelvic ultrasound scan revealed normal ovaries and uterus with an endometrium of 3 mm in thickness. The patient was reassured, but decided to see how she was without HRT. Her night sweats did not recur and she decided to remain off HRT.

COMMENTARY

There is a strong association between the menopause and the development of osteoporosis, with the main aetiological agent being the sudden fall in circulating oestrogens. Consequently, in situations where oestrogen levels are maintained, such as late menopause, obesity and in polycystic ovarian syndrome, the risk is lessened. Exercise helps to decrease bone loss following the menopause, whilst smokers have been found to have a lower bone density than non-smokers. Bone loss starts gradually over the decade leading up to the menopause, but afterwards the fall in density increases significantly. Without any hormone replacement, there may be a loss of 30–40% of bone mass before the age of 65 years (Hausen *et al*, 1991) (**Q1: true = D, E; false = A, B, C**).

When advising patients on whether to take HRT, particularly when they have no menopausal symptoms, it is helpful to ascertain the woman's menopausal status. With regular menstrual cycles, it is unlikely that her natural oestrogen levels would be low. Elevated levels of FSH (>15 IU l^{-1}) may be useful and indicate the woman is climacteric. If the levels indicate menopausal status, you should counsel the woman on her particular risk factors for developing osteoporosis, as well as considering the more general advantages and disadvantages of taking HRT (**Q2**).

You should be concerned about starting HRT in a woman with prolonged and irregular bleeding. Endometrial cancer is a concern in a woman with such symptoms at this age and, although dysfunctional bleeding is the most likely diagnosis, you should exclude more serious disease before commencing HRT (endometrial cancer is discussed in case 43). In addition, hormone treatment may mask the symptoms and signs of endometrial cancer. Ultrasonography may be useful in excluding malignancy if the endometrium is less than 6 mm thick; however, this is a more useful test in older women as around the menopause many women with normal endometrium have a thicker measurement. Endometrial biopsy should be undertaken, and may be achieved with an outpatient sampling device (**Q3**).

A diagnosis of simple cystic hyperplasia is a potential problem in this situation. It is very unlikely to progress to invasive cancer, with a risk of under 5%, and does not require hysterectomy. Management depends on symptoms and, in this case, progestogen therapy would probably reverse the hyperplasia as well as regulating the cycles. However, it is probably wise to perform a complete curettage of the uterus to include severe hyperplasia – both architectural and cytological (**Q4: true = D, E; false = A, B, C**).

It is always difficult to justify continuation of any treatment being used prophylactically when the patient experiences unpleasant side-effects. However, in the case of HRT the therapeutic long-term benefits may justify certain inconvenience. As this woman's main reason for taking HRT was the prevention of osteoporosis, an assessment of her bone mineral density was a sensible approach (**Q5**).

There are various methods of assessing BMD. Plain radiography, magnetic resonance imaging and computed tomography may all give information on bone mass, but perhaps the most widely used correct method is dual-photon absorptiometry. It gives a reliable assessment of both cortical and trabecular bone density (American College of Physicians, 1984) and is particularly useful in monitoring the need for treatment as well as its effect over a number of years. Ultrasonography is not particularly useful for assessing bone mineral content (**Q6: true = A, C, D; false = B**).

The aetiology of vasomotor symptoms is uncertain. Whilst oestrogen replacement is effective in alleviating them, there are certain situations in which oestrogen levels are low or are falling, such as in primary ovarian failure, when they do not occur. Similarly, there is poor correlation between gonadotrophin levels and the occurrence of such symptoms (**Q7**).

Whilst the development of a breast cyst would not be an indication for stopping HRT, one could understand the woman's anxieties about continuing with it. Other options for prevention of osteoporosis would include avoidance of risk factors such as smoking and anorexia, as well as regular exercise and possibly calcium supplements. In addition, she may be prepared to take tibolone to control her hot flushes and night sweats and avoid taking oestrogen (tibolone therapy is discussed further in case 43) (**Q8**).

REFERENCES

American College of Physicians. Radiologic methods to evaluate bone mineral content. *Ann Intern Med* 1984; **100**, 908–911.

Hausen MA, Overgaard K, Riis BJ, Christiansen C. Role of peak bone mass and bone loss in post menopausal osteoporosis. *BMJ* 1991; **303**: 961–964.

FACTS YOU SHOULD HAVE LEARNT . . .

▶ Management of the menopause
▶ Prevention and monitoring of osteoporosis
▶ Management of simple cystic hyperplasia of the endometrium

CASE 45

Prolapse

A 60-year-old woman attended the outpatient clinic complaining of constant low back pain associated with urinary frequency and a feeling of incomplete bladder emptying. She often leaked urine on standing following micturition although she did not complain of any other incontinence.

Q1: **Which of the following conditions should be included in your differential diagnosis?**
A: Recurrent urinary tract infections.
B: Ovarian cancer.
C: Constipation.
D: Uterovaginal prolapse.

On examination, the abdomen was soft with no tenderness or masses noted. On pelvic assessment, there was a large cystocele with cervical descent almost to the vaginal introitus. There was a moderate rectocele. The uterus was normal in size and mobile, and there was no evidence of an ovarian mass.

Q2: **How would you counsel the woman?**

After discussion, the patient opted for surgical management of the prolapse. She was concerned about her urinary symptoms and wished to be reassured that they would be better after the operation. In addition, she mentioned that her mother had died from ovarian cancer and she wondered whether her ovaries could be removed at the time of surgery. A decision was made to perform a laparoscopically assisted vaginal hysterectomy.

Q3: **Which of the following investigations would you perform?**
A: Urine culture.
B: Subtracted cystometry.
C: Intravenous pyelography.
D: Residual volume.

Q4: **What other surgical procedures could you have considered?**

The operation proceeded without complication, but 12 hours after the procedure the patient complained of feeling faint. She was restless and was found to have a pulse of 105 beats per minute (bpm) with a blood pressure of 60/30 mmHg. Abdominal tenderness was noted with generalized guarding.

Q5: What should be your immediate management?

On removing the vaginal pack there was no blood in the vagina and the suture line was intact. This was taken down and, on inspecting the pedicles, there was a sudden onset of heavy blood loss through the purse-string suture. On further exploration this appeared to be arising from the right infundibulopelvic ligament. It was not possible to obtain haemostasis via the vaginal route and consequently a Pfannenstiel incision was made and the bleeding was controlled by suturing the vessel. The estimated blood loss was 3 litres and the patient was given 6 units of blood. The anaesthetist wished to maintain assisted ventilation overnight and the patient was transferred to the intensive care unit.

Q6: What were the anaesthetist's concerns and what were the reasons for admission to intensive care?

The woman was extubated on the following morning and went back to the general ward 12 hours later. She made a full recovery and went home 1 week later.

When seen for a follow-up visit 6 weeks later, she complained of persistent right-sided abdominal pain which radiated around to her back. She had no other symptoms; she was passing urine normally and had a daily bowel action. There had been no significant vaginal discharge or bleeding. Examination revealed tenderness in the right iliac fossa and right loin.

Q7: Which of the following should be included in your differential diagnosis?
A: Gallstones.
B: Irritable bowel.
C: Ureteric obstruction.
D: Appendicitis.

An ultrasound scan confirmed a right hydronephritis with marked dilatation of the ureter to about the level of the pelvic brim, where there appeared to be an obstruction. A cystoscopy was performed and an attempt was made to pass a stent up the ureter from the bladder in the hope of passing the obstruction, but this was unsuccessful. The ureter was approached abdominally and was found to be narrowed close to the pelvic inlet. Following mobilization the obstruction was bypassed by means of division above and below, and reanastomosis was achieved. The ureteric stent was removed via a cystoscope 1 week later after an intravenous pyelogram (IVP) had confirmed satisfactory function.

Q8: How would you manage her follow-up?

COMMENTARY

The symptoms of urinary frequency, low back pain and a feeling of incomplete bladder emptying may be associated with recurrent urinary tract infections as well as uterovaginal prolapse. Bladder symptoms may also result from extrinsic pressure due to pelvic tumours such as ovarian cysts and uterine fibroids, and these may cause back pain. Constipation would not cause such urinary symptoms (**Q1: true = A, B, D; false = C**). Having examined the patient, she was found to have a significant prolapse involving the anterior and posterior vaginal walls as well as the uterus. In counselling the woman you should indicate the cause of her symptoms and the possible ways of alleviating them. There are two possible treatments, namely surgery or the use of a vaginal pessary. In a 60-year-old woman one would favour surgical correction of the prolapse. Clearly there are risks and complications of surgery and the patient may consider that her symptoms do not justify this. If she opts for an operation, it is important to ascertain whether or not she is sexually active as any prolapse repair is a compromise between minimizing the risk of recurrence and the retention of a functional vagina. In addition, it is important to obtain consent to enable a decision on the exact surgery performed to be made at the time, as assessment of the prolapse is much more accurate when the woman is anaesthetized (**Q2**).

The urinary symptoms are likely to be corrected by a repair operation, but you should take a more detailed history of bladder function. In the absence of any other symptoms such as urgency, incontinence and significant nocturia the authors would not recommend subtracted cystometry. Urine culture would be mandatory and if this were negative an IVP would not be necessary. A residual measurement after micturition would be helpful to confirm adequate bladder emptying (**Q3: true = A, D; false = B, C**).

With a history of her mother dying from ovarian cancer, the patient's request for removal of her ovaries is reasonable as her risk of developing ovarian cancer is of the order of 5%. The options would be to perform a laparoscopically assisted vaginal hysterectomy with repair, or to perform a vaginal hysterectomy in the usual way and take the ovaries out via the vagina. It is often possible to perform the latter procedure, but if one is not successful it is necessary to perform a laparotomy via a Pfannenstiel incision after completing the vaginal surgery. In this case, the ovaries were freed laparoscopically using a stapling device (**Q4**).

On being faced with a patient in the condition described 12 hours after surgery, the diagnosis is one of haemoperitoneum necessitating urgent correction of the bleeding. Your immediate management should include rapid infusion of colloid to expand the circulating volume, and urgent cross-matching and transfusion. The patient should be taken back to theatre immediately. During a standard vaginal hysterectomy one would hope that bleeding would be revealed vaginally as the pedicles are kept extraperitoneally. However, this is not always the case, although exploration through the vagina is usually successful in resolving the problem. In this case a laparotomy was necessary, with a 6-unit blood transfusion (**Q5**).

After operation, the level of continued care will depend on the need for further resuscitation, monitoring and physiological support. Although the bleeding has been stopped, a pathophysiological legacy will persist. Major system ischaemia (cerebral, myocardial, renal) may have resulted from the period of hypotension, hypothermia, anaemia and transfusion of stored blood. Bleeding may resume due to the lack of coagulation factors and platelets. Admission to intensive care with continued ventilation may be advised. Such treatment would ensure optimum oxygenation by stabilizing the respiratory system, minimizing the work of breathing for the compromised myocardium, and allowing normothermia to be achieved. At the same time continued monitoring would facilitate evaluation and further treatment, blood component administration, inotropic cardiovascular support, additional fluids and diuretics. Once homeostasis has been achieved spontaneous ventilation could be recommenced (**Q6**).

After initial recovery and during the following few weeks, a history of right-sided abdominal pain radiating to the back should raise the possibility of ureteric damage. Whilst gallstones and irritable bowel may also cause such symptoms, this new problem is more likely to be related to the recent surgery. Appendicitis does not present in this chronic manner (**Q7: true = A, B, C; false = D**). Having made the diagnosis of ureteric obstruction, referral to an appropriate urological surgeon is essential as the initial attempt at relieving the obstruction is the most likely to be effective. Following successful reanastomosis, it is important to ensure that the function remains normal, and you should repeat an IVP approximately 3 months after the reanastamosis (**Q8**).

FACTS YOU SHOULD HAVE LEARNT . . .

▶ **The management of uterovaginal prolapse**
▶ **The management of postoperative bleeding**
▶ **The ongoing support of the shocked patient**

CASE 46

Urinary incontinence

A 36-year-old woman presented with a history of increasing leakage of urine since her last child was born 2 years previously. The leakage occurred mainly on exertion but also on coughing and sneezing. She had no symptoms of urinary urgency or frequency and rarely had to go to the toilet at night. She thought that the bladder emptied completely on voiding. Examination did not reveal any abdominal masses, but on vaginal assessment she had a moderate cystocele and rectocele with minimal uterocervical descent. The uterus was normal in size and there was no ovarian enlargement. Urinary incontinence was not demonstrated initially, but 1 hour after consuming 1 litre of water some leakage was observed on coughing. She subsequently voided 400 ml of urine and the residual volume was 10 ml.

Q1: What is the most likely diagnosis?
   A: Detrusor instability.
   B: Genuine stress incontinence.
   C: Overflow incontinence.
   D: Neurogenic bladder.
   E: Cystitis

Q2: How would you manage the problem?

Following the appropriate investigation, a diagnosis of genuine stress incontinence was made.

Q3: Which of the following treatments would be appropriate options?
   A: Oxybutynin hydrochloride.
   B: Pelvic floor physiotherapy.
   C: Intermittent self-catheterization.
   D: Oestrogen vagina cream.
   E: Colposuspension.

After informed discussion, the patient considered that further physiotherapy was unlikely to be beneficial as she had done pelvic floor exercises regularly since the birth of her last child. The incontinence was preventing her from going out socially and, whilst she was undecided regarding further pregnancies, she was prepared to accept that if she had another child it would be sensible to undergo elective Caesarean section. She elected to undergo surgery.

Q4: Which of the following factors should influence your choice of operation:

A: The patient's age.
B: The presence of vaginal prolapse.
C: The patient's weight.
D: Surgical morbidity.
E: The presence of urinary infection.

The woman underwent a Burch colposuspension operation with posterior colpoperineorrhaphy. She made a satisfactory recovery, but was unable to void completely after clamping of the suprapubic catheter. Two weeks after surgery, the residual volume after micturition varied between 250 and 400 ml.

Q5: What are the different treatment options you could use to deal with this problem?

The post-micturition residual volume fell to around 100 ml during the week after treatment. The suprapubic catheter was removed and the patient went home. At the follow-up visit 6 weeks later, she reported complete control with no incontinence. She did have to strain and thought that bladder emptying took longer than before surgery. She often had the need to go to the toilet soon after the previous visit. A measurement of residual volume was 250 ml.

Q6: Which of the following alternatives would you recommend?
A: Discharge from the clinic.
B: Admission for investigations.
C: Reassurance with follow-up in 3 months.
D: Subtracted cystometry.

Six months later, the patient had maintained total urinary continence with normal flow rates and satisfactory bladder emptying.

COMMENTARY

Urinary incontinence may be classified in the following way:
- Genuine stress incontinence.
- Detrusor instability.
- Overflow incontinence.
- True incontinence (fistula).
- Neurogenic incontinence.
- Psychogenic incontinence.
- Congenital incontinence (persistent).

The first two are the commonest causes in adult gynaecological practice. In this case, the most likely diagnosis is genuine stress incontinence, although there is a significant chance that the patient has detrusor instability or a mixed picture of both diagnoses (Jarvis, 1990), although urinary infection should always be excluded (**Q1: true = B; false = A, C, D, E**).

It is clearly important to make a correct diagnosis before embarking on treatment and the patient should undergo subtracted cystometry. This involves the passage of a urethral catheter into the bladder with a pressure transducer alongside it and another pressure transducer inserted into the rectum. The bladder is filled via the catheter, usually with sterile saline, at about 100 ml per minute. The rectal pressure, recording the intraperitoneal pressure, is subtracted from the intravesical pressure to give the detrusor pressure. You should also record the maximum bladder capacity and the residual urine volume following micturition. The patient should stand and cough at some stage during the procedure to see whether this produces detrusor activity. In the case discussed, you should have expected no rise in detrusor pressure during filling, with a capacity of 400–500 ml and a residual volume of less than 50 ml. You may not necessarily demonstrate incontinence even if there is a sphincter weakness and, if this is so, you should perform videocystourethrography which involves radiological imaging of the bladder and urethra using an image intensifier whilst a cystometrogram is performed (Bates *et al*, 1970). This will help to outline the shape and position of the bladder neck and in the case discussed should have confirmed the diagnosis (**Q2**).

The management options for genuine stress incontinence include physiotherapy, possibly using weighted vaginal cones to assess muscle tone, periurethral collagen injections to increase urethral resistance, local vaginal oestrogen cream in postmenopausal women, and surgery to elevate the bladder neck. Oxybutynin hydrochloride is an anticholinergic agent used in the management of detrusor instability, whilst intermittent self-catheterization is reserved for individuals with voiding difficulties. The choice of treatment will be influenced by the patient's perception of the problem, how much it interferes with her life, as well as her wish for further pregnancies. The purpose of surgery is elevation of the bladder neck that results in increased urethral resistance to bladder emptying by increasing the length of the urethra which reduces the diameter and reduces the closing pressure. Such elevation would undoubtedly be reversed by a subsequent vaginal delivery, and you should anticipate a recurrence of the problem in these circumstances (**Q3: true = B, E; false = A, C, D**).

There are numerous operations for genuine stress incontinence, divided into abdominal, vaginal and combined procedures. In general, you should advocate the operation with the highest success rate. However, there is a trade-off between success and complications of surgery, and the latter may be increased considerably in obese patients particularly when an abdominal approach is undertaken. In elderly patients with atrophic tissues there may not be sufficient laxity in the anterior vaginal wall to achieve satisfactory elevation by means of an abdominal procedure. Similarly, the presence of prolapse may influence one's decision, although it is important to consider the patient's main symptoms. It is possible to deal with anterior vaginal wall prolapse via an abdominal procedure. Vaginal procedures are quicker and technically easier than other operations and are associated with less surgical morbidity. However, the long-term results are generally less successful (**Q4: true = A, B, C, D; false = E**).

In this case, the authors would have favoured a Burch colposuspension operation. It carries the best long-term success rate, although it may be associated with considerable morbidity. Postoperative voiding disorders are perhaps the most important, but also vaginal prolapse particularly of the posterior wall and dyspareunia may occur. The patient discussed above had a rectocele and hence this was repaired at the time of surgery. There is a risk of developing detrusor instability after any procedure for genuine stress incontinence.

Unfortunately, this patient developed outflow obstruction after the bladder neck had been elevated. The risks of this are overflow incontinence, urinary stasis causing recurrent infections, and subsequent ascending infection and renal damage. Urethral dilatation is often carried out in this situation and in the case discussed seems to have been helpful (**Q5**). It was not curative, as the residual volume had risen after discharge from hospital to 250 ml at the follow-up visit. The patient should have been admitted at this stage (**Q6: true = B; false = A, C, D**). The options would now have been intermittent self-catheterization or complete drainage and rest of the bladder for a period of time, usually 1 week. Following this, clamping of the catheter should have been performed combined with cholinergic therapy to try to induce detrusor activity. In this case, it was successful and intermittent self-catheterization was not required.

REFERENCES

Bates CP, Whiteside CG, Turner-Warwick RT. Synchronous cine/pressure/flow/cystourethrography with special reference to stress and urge incontinence. *Br J Urol* 1970; **42**: 714–723.

Jarvis GJ. The place of urodynamic investigation. In: Jarvis GJ (ed.) *Female Urinary Incontinence*, pp 15–20. London: Royal College of Obstetricians and Gynaecologists, 1990.

FACTS YOU SHOULD HAVE LEARNT . . .

- ▶ The investigation and classification of urinary incontinence
- ▶ The management of genuine stress incontinence
- ▶ The management of outflow obstruction

CASE 47

Vulval carcinoma

A 77-year-old woman was referred by her general practitioner to the gynaecology outpatient clinic with a long history of vulval irritation. She had used various creams with limited effect, but was concerned because of a recent episode of fresh bleeding followed by brown staining of her underwear for 2 weeks. She was overweight and abdominal examination was unremarkable. On inspection of the vulva there was a raised lesion, about 1.5 cm in diameter that looked like a carcinoma. The rest of the vulva was rather atrophic and vaginal examination was otherwise unremarkable.

QI: What would be your immediate management?

Wide local excision of the lesion confirmed a well-differentiated squamous cell carcinoma with the margins well clear of the tumour.

Q2: Which of the following would you recommend?
A: No further treatment.
B: Simple vulvectomy.
C: Radical vulvectomy with separate groin incisions.
D: Radical vulvectomy with connecting incisions.

After appropriate counselling, she was readmitted for radical vulvectomy. This was performed using separate groin incisions and was uncomplicated. An indwelling catheter was left at the end of the procedure along with a suction drain in each groin wound.

Q3: In what circumstances would you carry out pelvic lymphadenectomy?

Q4: What instructions would you give to the ward staff for postoperative care?

On the second postoperative day, the suction drain fell out on the right side. The left-sided drain continued to accumulate more than 100 ml of fluid each day until the eighth day, when it was removed. The groin wound remained intact and the vulva healed well after some initial oedema and bruising. The patient passed urine normally after the catheter was removed on the seventh day.

Histological examination of the specimen revealed no residual vulval tumour. Two of the lymph glands from the left side contained metastatic tumour.

The patient was treated with a course of external-beam pelvic radiotherapy which started 2 weeks after she was discharged home. She received 4000 cGy in 20 fractions over a period of 4 weeks.

Q5: What are the common complications of pelvic radiotherapy?

The patient was reviewed in the outpatient clinic 2 months after completion of radiotherapy. She complained of a tender swelling in her right groin.

Q6: Which of the following should be included in the differential diagnosis?
A: Femoral artery aneurysm.
B: Lymphocyst.
C: Femoral hernia.
D: Recurrent tumour.

Needle aspiration confirmed the presence of a lymphocyst. Examination was otherwise normal and arrangements were made to review her in 3 months.

Q7: How would you manage the lymphocyst?

At her next visit, the lymphocyst had filled up again although it was less swollen than before. It was causing less discomfort than previously and the patient did not wish to have it aspirated. There was no sign of any tumour recurrence.

Q8: What is the long-term morbidity associated with radical vulvectomy?

Three months later an irregular lesion was noted on the left side of the vulva, approximately 1 cm in diameter. A small biopsy taken in the clinic confirmed recurrent tumour.

Q9: Which of the following would you recommend?
A: Chemotherapy.
B: Iridium implants.
C: Wide local excision.
D: Laser vaporization.
E: Immunotherapy.

The excision margins were clear of tumour and the patient recovered well. Follow-up over the following 5 years was satisfactory and, whilst the lymphocyst remained, she did not find it a major inconvenience.

COMMENTARY

When you are clinically suspicious of a vulval tumour, it is imperative that the lesion is biopsied as a matter of some urgency. In the presence of a well-circumscribed simple lesion it is appropriate to perform a wide local excision as this would be adequate treatment whether the lesion turned out to be benign or the histology report confirmed a malignant melanoma (**Q1**).

The decision regarding further management should be based on the type of tumour, the depth of invasion and the general medical condition of the patient. In the case of a squamous cell carcinoma with a depth of invasion greater than 1 mm below the basement membrane, you should recommend radical vulvectomy if the woman were medically fit enough to undergo it. In stage I disease, such a procedure may be undertaken through separate groin incisions (Monaghan, 1990). The advantage of this approach is the markedly improved primary healing achieved compared with the butterfly incision, without any apparent decreased survival (**Q2: true = C; false = A, B, D**).

There are very few circumstances in which you should advocate pelvic lymphadenectomy for this disease. Homesley et al (1986) showed that the use of pelvic radiotherapy in patients with positive groin nodes gave a statistically significant improvement in survival compared with pelvic lymphadenectomy, with similar morbidity in both groups. The only indication to perform pelvic lymphadenectomy would be in a young woman with positive groin nodes at frozen section who wished to retain her reproductive potential (**Q3**).

Following surgery, you should instruct the ward staff to keep the vulval area meticulously clean without using any irritant fluids. The groin drains should be left *in situ* until they drain less than 100 ml over a 24-hour period, and the catheter should be left *in situ* for about 5–7 days to aid skin healing. Mobilization is extremely important as the risk of thromboembolism is great and prophylaxis with subcutaneous heparin and anti-embolism stockings should be employed. Pneumatic boots should be used during the procedure (**Q4**).

Following pelvic irradiation, the main short-term morbidity relates to bladder and bowel function. Cystitis with urinary frequency is common, as is proctitis and diarrhoea. Problems usually start a fortnight after the commencement of treatment, with a similar lag period after completion of radiotherapy. Longer term bladder and bowel morbidity may occur with a small volume bladder causing frequency and urgency and bowel strictures causing subacute obstruction. Both urinary and faecal fistula may occasionally follow radiotherapy treatment. The other significant risk of postoperative pelvic irradiation after radical vulvectomy is the risk of chronic lymphoedema of the lower limbs causing considerable swelling, discomfort and even ulceration (**Q5**).

The most likely cause of a groin swelling 2 months after treatment would be a lymphocyst, with recurrent tumour being unlikely so early in a well-differentiated carcinoma managed with surgery and radiotherapy. Whilst femoral artery aneurysm and hernia may occur, there is no particular reason why they should develop at this time (**Q6: true = B; false = A, C, D**).

The management of a lymphocyst may be difficult and is largely dependent on the symptoms it is causing. It is possible to keep aspirating it, but recurrence is inevitable and the only permanent treatment is surgical. One rarely has to revert to surgery unless the cyst is of very large volume (**Q7**).

The long-term morbidity following radical vulvectomy is frequently underrated. Lymphocysts and chronic oedema of the lower limb are not uncommon. Femoral nerve damage causing irritating paraesthesia over the front of the thigh (L1, 2) may occur. Chronic urinary infections may result from urethral damage, and incontinence can occur. Misdirection of the urinary stream may be troublesome. Significant distortion of the vulva is inevitable and this may cause considerable sexual dysfunction. The other major problem is that perineal support is lost and a resultant high risk of prolapse, particularly of the posterior vaginal wall (**Q8**).

The management of recurrent disease is dependent on its extent and location as well as what previous treatment has been used. Local recurrence is best treated by wide excision, assuming this is possible without compromising bladder or bowel function. If this is a risk, then iridium implants may be used to shrink the recurrence. Chemotherapy and laser vaporization are not recommended (**Q9: true = B, C; false = A, D, E**) and no immunotherapy is currently available.

REFERENCES

Homesley HD, Brundy BN, Sedlis A, Adcock L. Radiation therapy versus pelvic node resection for carcinoma of the vulva with positive groin nodes. *Obstet Gynecol* 1986, **68**: 733–740.

Monaghan JM. Management of vulval carcinoma. In: Shepherd J, Monaghan JM (eds) *Clinical Gynaecological Oncology*, 2nd edn, p 140–167. London: Blackwell Scientific Publications, 1990.

FACTS YOU SHOULD HAVE LEARNT . . .

▶ **The management of vulval carcinoma**
▶ **The complications of radical vulvectomy**
▶ **The complications of pelvic irradiation**

CASE 48

Vulval pruritus

A 47-year-old woman attended her general practitioner's surgery complaining of constant vulval itching for the previous 2 weeks. She had been having problems sleeping at night and the only relief she could obtain was from tepid baths. She was having regular menstrual cycles with no abnormal bleeding and had had a recent negative cervical smear. Examination revealed a generally reddened vulva with patches of raised white skin on both labia majora. The vagina and cervix looked healthy, and there was a small amount of white discharge. Pelvic assessment was otherwise normal.

Q1: Which of the following should be included in the differential diagnosis?
A: Candidal infection.
B: Acute genital herpes.
C: Lichen sclerosus.
D: Molluscum contagiosum.
E: Lichen planus.

Her general practitioner gave her a prescription for Canesten-HC cream and advised her to apply it to the sore areas twice daily for 2 weeks. He arranged to review her then.

She gained a little relief over the first few days but unfortunately this was only transient. The appearance of the vulva was unchanged.

Her general practitioner referred her to the gynaecology outpatient clinic, where the findings were unchanged.

Q2: How would you manage the patient?

Two biopsies were taken from the affected area. She was advised to use clobetasol propionate (0.05%) (Dermovate) cream sparingly over the next 6 weeks when she was to be reviewed with the result of the biopsies taken in the clinic.

Q3: How would you advise her to use the cream?

Q4: What are the risks of strong steroid creams?

When the patient next attended, her symptoms had improved dramatically and the vulva looked less red than before. The patches of white skin on both labia majora persisted. The biopsies from these areas both showed lichen sclerosus. In one of them, there was an area of vulval intraepithelial neoplasia grade III (VIN III) extending to an excision margin.

Q5:   Which of the following would you recommend?
   A: Simple vulvectomy.
   B: Further use of clobetasol propionate (Dermovate) cream.
   C: Wide excision of the white areas of skin.
   D: Radical vulvectomy.
   E: Microscopic assessment of the vulva.

At the time of vulvoscopy, the areas of white skin on both labia became much more densely white with application of acetic acid. In addition, there was some mosaic patterning on the right side. The remaining vulval skin did not alter its appearance in response to acetic acid.

Q6:   How would you manage this situation?

The patient was admitted as a day case and underwent wide local excision of both patches of white skin. She made a good recovery and was seen 2 weeks later to discuss the histology report. This confirmed widespread lichen sclerosus adjacent to areas of VIN III. On the biopsy from the right labia majora there was a small bud of VIN III breaching the basement membrane to a depth of 0.5 mm. The lichen sclerosus extended to all excision margins, but the VIN III was completely excised.

Q7:   What is the relationship between lichen sclerosus and invasive vulval cancer?

Q8:   How would you manage the patient now?

The patient was reviewed in the colposcopy clinic 6 months later. She had not needed any further treatment for vulval pruritus. On colposcopic assessment, the vulva had healed well and there were no areas of acetowhite epithelium.

Q9:   What follow-up would you recommend?

COMMENTARY

Vulval pruritus is a very common complaint. Whilst it is more common in older women, it can affect all age groups. Aetiological factors include non-neoplastic disorders of the vulva, other dermatoses and infections. In this case, the differential diagnosis included candidal infection, lichen sclerosus and lichen planus. Acute genital herpes is an acute blistering eruption which causes marked swelling of the vulva, whilst molluscum contagiosum causes small blisters not usually seen on the vulva (**Q1: true = A, C, E; false = B, D**).

The initial management will be influenced by the appearance of the vulva and whether or not the clinician considers that a biopsy should be performed. The advantages of a biopsy are a more precise diagnosis and also the exclusion of underlying malignancy. Transient vulval pruritus in the absence of any worrying physical signs is very common and the general practitioner could not be criticized for giving a course of clotrimazole cream containing hydrocortisone (Canesten-HC) initially. Failure to respond to this resulted in an appropriate hospital referral, where biopsies were taken and stronger steroid cream prescribed. Outpatient biopsies are simple to take with local anaesthetic and the use of a ring biopsy to remove a small core of vulval skin. Bleeding can usually be controlled by direct pressure although a suture may sometimes be required. It was reasonable to prescribe symptomatic treatment in view of the non-specific vulval appearance before obtaining the histology report (**Q2**). One may question the use of such a strong steroid cream at this stage. The authors would recommend the application of a small amount of clobetasol propionate (Dermovate) cream rubbed well into the sore areas twice a day for 2 weeks followed by once daily for 2 weeks, and then once on alternate days for a final 2 weeks (**Q3**).

Strong steroid creams are absorbed into the circulation and may result in Cushing's syndrome. They must be used sparingly and for only limited time periods as prolonged use may result in hypoplasia of the dermis and epidermis. They may also aggravate local infections and can cause contact dermatitis (**Q4**).

The occurrence of VIN III on the biopsies, particularly incompletely excised, necessitated a more detailed examination of the vulva with a colposcope. Whilst further surgical treatment may have been indicated, this should have been performed only in the light of more detailed assessment. Microscopic examination is less useful in vulval disease than on the cervix, as keratin interferes with the response to acetic acid and vessel changes are less commonly noted. It is, however, helpful in assessing the extent of the abnormality as well as excluding invasive disease (**Q5: true = E; false = A, B, C, D**).

The natural history of VIN is less well understood than that of cervical intraepithelial neoplasia (CIN). The risk of progression to invasive disease is much less on the vulva, and the treatment of VIN is considerably more complicated and mutilating than that of CIN. For these reasons, you should be much more conservative in the management of patients with VIN. In the case described, there were two well-defined areas of abnormality with normal skin elsewhere. The management of this situation would be influenced by this finding as well as by the fact that these two areas of skin were responsible for the woman's symptoms. In addition, the original biopsy showed VIN III and you should therefore have recommended wide local excision of the two areas (**Q6**).

The histology of the excised skin confirmed VIN III with lichen sclerosis, and there was a small area of invasive vulval cancer on the right side. There has been considerable interest in the relationship between lichen sclerosis and carcinoma of the vulva. The former is relatively common whilst the latter is an uncommon tumour. Lichen sclerosis has been reported in association with vulval cancer (Ansink *et al*, 1994). Whether there is a causal relationship between the two conditions is certainly not proven (**Q7**).

The findings of an area of invasive disease is extremely important from the point of view of the patient's management. Fortunately, there does not appear to be any risk of nodal metastases in lesions invading to a depth of less than 1 mm below the basement membrane and wide local excision should be curative (Wilkinson, 1985) (**Q8**). However, because VIN is a multifocal condition, the patient is at risk of developing it elsewhere on her vulva. You should therefore recommend long-term microscopic follow-up of this patient with annual assessments at a minimum. As lichen sclerosis is an autoimmune condition you should check a full blood count looking for evidence of pernicious anaemia (low haemoglobin and elevated mean corpuscular volume). Thyroid function tests should also be performed and many would advocate an autoimmune screen to assess the presence of autoimmune antibodies in the patient's serum (**Q9**).

REFERENCES

Ansink AC, Krul MR, De Weger RA et al. Human papilloma virus, lichen sclerosus and squamous cell carcinoma of the vulva: detection and prognostic significance. *Gynecol Oncol* 1994; **52**: 180–184.

Wilkinson EJ. Superficial invasive cancer of the vulva. *Clin Obstet Gynecol* 1985; **28**: 188–195.

FACTS YOU SHOULD HAVE LEARNT . . .

▶ The causes and management of vulval pruritus
▶ The assessment and management of vulval intraepithelial neoplasia

CASE 49

Virilization

A 53-year-old married P2 + 0 Caucasian woman presented to the gynaecology outpatient clinic with a 2-year history of increasing body hair and worsening frontal balding (see Figure 4). On direct questioning she had noticed a deepening in her voice and an increase in facial hair but no increase in acne and seborrhoea. At the age of 42 years she had undergone the menopause. She had a past medical history of hypertension, myxoedema and hypercholesterolaemia, all of which were treated adequately and appropriately with lisinopril (5 mg daily) thyroxine (75 μg daily) and pravastatin (10 mg daily) respectively. On examination, the blood pressure was 150/90 mmHg. She had marked frontal balding with a Ferriman–Galwey score of 28. The body mass index was 27, there were no

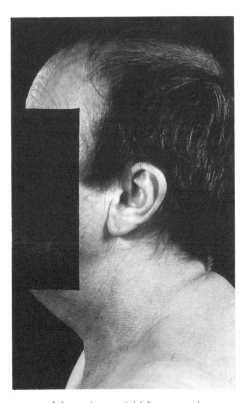

Figure 4   The appearance of the patient on initial presentation.

abdominal striae and a normal body fat distribution was noted. There was no goitre and her breasts were normal with no galactorrhoea. The abdomen was soft and non-tender and there were no masses palpable. The rest of the examination was unremarkable apart from clitoromegaly (3 cm).

QI: Which of the following statements are correct?

A: This woman had a premature menopause.

B: All the medications this woman is taking would be safe in early pregnancy.

C: The woman has Cushing's syndrome until proven otherwise.

D: The woman is at high risk of coronary artery disease.

E: Cholesterol is the precursor for all hormones produced by the endogenous enzyme pathways of steroidogenesis.

The results of hormonal investigations were as follows: testosterone 33.3 nmol l^{-1}, androstenedione 19.5 nmol l^{-1}, 17-hydroxyprogesterone (17-OHP) 9.9 nmol l^{-1}, dihydroepiandrostenedione sulphate (DHEAS) 4.4 μmol l^{-1}, follicle stimulating hormone (FSH) 48.9 IU l^{-1}, luteinizing hormone (LH) 29.2 IU l^{-1}, prolactin 450 mIU l^{-1}.

Q2: What is your interpretation of these results and what should be your next investigation?

Q3: What condition must be excluded in this case?

An abdominal ultrasound scan was normal. Abdominal computed tomography (CT) showed no enlargement of the adrenal glands and no other masses. The 2-day dexamethasone suppression test revealed the results shown in Table 3:

TABLE 3 RESULTS OF DEXAMETHASONE SUPPRESSION TEST

Time	Cortisol (nmol l^{-1})	Testosterone (nmol l^{-1})	17-OHP (nmol l^{-1})
Pretreatment	584	35.3	10.5
+12 hours	608	30.1	12.6
+24 hours	25	32.8	11.8
+36 hours	0	35.8	11.0
+48 hours	0	39.8	13.1

Q4: Which of the following about the dexamethasone suppression test results are correct?

A: Testosterone did not suppress, therefore it is most likely to be an ovarian tumour.

B: Cortisol did suppress, therefore Cushing's syndrome has been excluded.

C: 17-OHP did not suppress, therefore congenital adrenal hyperplasia has been excluded.

D: 17-OHP exhibited nyctohemeral variation.

E: The patient has Addison's disease at +48 hours

F: The patient is suffering from Nelson's syndrome

TABLE 4 RESULTS OF SELECTIVE VENOUS SAMPLING

Venous site	Testosterone (nmol l⁻¹)	Cortisol (nmol⁻¹)	Androstenedione (nmol l⁻¹)	DHEAS (nmol l⁻¹)
Right renal	26.7/24.1	577/648	25.8/23.0	4.0/3.6
Left renal	25.9/24.6	552/490	20.6/22.4	3.9/3.9
Left adrenal	36.1/24.6	679/565	38.0/23.4	4.4/4.0
Right adrenal	17.5/21.8	550/421	28.6/20.8	2.7/2.7
Inferior vena caval	24.3/21.9	495/474	20.2/20.0	1.7/2.7
Left ovarian	19.9/22.6	395/517	16.6/18.8	2.6/1.8
Right ovarian	261.0/20.4	376/407	286.0/25.2	3.0/3.1

Selective venous sampling was performed to localize the testosterone-secreting tumour. This procedure revealed the results shown in Table 4 (the numerator is the local nominated sample and the denominator is the peripheral blood sample taken at the same time).

Q5: Why is the androstenedione concentration raised in the right ovarian vein?

Q6: What is your interpretation of the result and what is your recommended treatment?

An uncomplicated abdominal total hysterectomy and bilateral salpingo-oöphorectomy was performed. The histology revealed a small benign hilar cell tumour 0.8 cm in diameter in the right ovary. The peritoneal washings obtained for cytological assessment were negative.

Q7: Would you give this woman oestrogen replacement therapy?

At the 6-week postoperative visit she was well but had stopped her oestrogen therapy because she had suffered headaches. The blood hormone levels were as follows: testosterone < 1.7 nmol l⁻¹, oestradiol < 25.0 pmol l⁻¹, FSH = 71.8 IU l⁻¹.

Q8: What manipulations with the oestrogen therapy may help with this side-effect?

Q9: What are the other common oestrogen side-effects?

COMMENTARY

This woman presented with a premature menopause which is currently defined as menopause before 45 years of age. In fact it should be treated clinically as secondary amenorrhoea. Thyroxine is essential in early pregnancy for myxoedematous women but the other two medications are contraindicated in early pregnancy. Angiotensin-converting enzyme inhibitors cause fetal and neonatal renal abnormalities and dysfunction associated with oligohydramnios and possibly skull defects. Any woman with hypertension and hirsutism should be considered to have Cushing's syndrome until proven otherwise, regardless of the apparent absence of clinical signs. This patient was at high risk of coronary artery disease because of the hypertension, myxoedema, hypercholesterolaemia and hyperandrogenaemia with hypooestrogenaemia. Cholesterol is the precursor for all steroid hormones (**Q1: true = A, C, D, E; false = B**).

The hormone investigations that must be performed include assessment of the androgens testosterone, androstenedione and DHEAS. The hormone precursor 17-OHP must be measured as levels are raised in congenital adrenal hyperplasia. The gonadotrophins FSH, LH and also prolactin should be measured to ensure that premature menopause is the correct diagnosis. These results indicate the possible presence of a testosterone-secreting tumour in either the ovary or the adrenal gland, and imaging techniques need to be employed to localize it. Ultrasonography and CT should be used to help but magnetic resonance imaging will improve the resolution (**Q2**).

Cushing's syndrome must be excluded with a 2-day dexamethasone suppression test (0.5 mg twice a day with estimations of cortisol, testosterone and 17-OHP at 0900 and 2100 hours) (**Q3**).

The testosterone did not suppress in the dexamethasone suppression test; therefore the raised testosterone levels were most likely to be due to an ovarian tumour. However, the cortisol levels were suppressed, so that Cushing's syndrome can be excluded. Generally, 17-OHP of adrenal origin will be suppressed by dexamethasone, excluding congenital adrenal hyperplasia. 17-OHP levels can be raised in polycystic ovary syndrome but usually the levels of 17-OHP originating from the ovary will not be suppressed. The diagnosis of congenital adrenal hyperplasia is made by an adrenocorticotrophic hormone (ACTH) stimulation test. In this test result, the 17-OHP did not exhibit nyctohemeral or diurnal variation and thus the patient had neither Addison's disease nor Nelson's syndrome (**Q4: true = A, B; false = C, D, E, F**).

This patient required selective venous sampling to localize the testosterone-secreting tumour. The level of androstenedione was increased in the right ovarian vein because it is the precursor steroid of testosterone synthesis. The enzyme 17-ketosteroid reductase converts androstenedione to testosterone by reducing the ketone bond to an alcohol on C17 in the D ring of the steroid molecule. Androstenedione can also be converted to oestrone by the action of the enzyme aromatase (**Q5**).

The woman had a testosterone-secreting tumour in the right ovary. She required an abdominal total hysterectomy and bilateral salpingo-oöphorectomy. A right salpingo-oöphorectomy would have been adequate surgical treatment in a younger woman who wished to preserve her fertility. Peritoneal washings should be obtained for cytological assessment to stage the disease should the tumour be malignant, although this is unusual. You should always remember that it is essential to take peritoneal washings in all cases of ovarian cysts and tumours (**Q6**).

It is essential that this woman should be given oestrogen replacement therapy as it will help to reverse her adverse lipid profile and thus reduce her risk of myocardial infarction. It will help with the regression of the virilization process and hirsutism. She was probably not at great risk of osteoporosis as the testosterone stimulates osteoblast bone formation, rather than osteoclastic resorption, in the bone turnover equation. The only potential risk with long-term (more than 8–10 years) use of oestrogen replacement therapy is that of breast cancer, and at present it is not known whether this effect is causative or promoting. The route of oestrogen administration depends on patient preference to enhance compliance and cost. All methods are of proven efficacy (**Q7**). Whatever the route of administration chosen, the initial dose must be small with a long build-up to the recommended dose, as this woman is at risk of developing oestrogen-dependent side-effects. For the oral preparations you should initially prescribe oestradiol 1 mg at night every other night and then slowly increase the dose. If side-effects are reported, you should reduce the dose for 2 weeks and then recommence increasing the dose. Similarly with transdermal patches, you should start at 25 µg. Obviously this woman does not need a progestogen (**Q8**).

Other common side-effects with oestrogen therapy are mastalgia, weight gain and nausea. Again, the principles are the same: start with a low dose, use a formulation that you can manipulate, reassure your patient and wait for her body to develop tolerance. Weight gain is probably not attributable to oestrogen but more a symptom of well-being (**Q9**).

FACTS YOU SHOULD HAVE LEARNT . . .

- ▶ **The appropriate investigation of a patient with virilization**
- ▶ **The management of a patient with a raised testosterone level**
- ▶ **Side-effects of hormone replacement therapy**

CASE 50

Male subfertility

A couple presented with a history of primary subfertility. They had been trying to conceive for 2 years. Previously, the woman had used the oral contraceptive pill for 5 years. After stopping the pill, she had had regular menstrual cycles of 28 days. She had no past history of any operations and had never had any significant pelvic infection. Her husband was fit and healthy with no relevant illnesses or operations. They had intercourse approximately three times each week without any problem.

Examination of the woman revealed normal breasts and pelvic organs with a small, mobile uterus and no adnexal masses. Her husband had normal-sized testes with no evidence of any hernia or varicocele.

Q1: How would you counsel the couple?

Q2: What investigations would you recommend?

The woman's hormonal investigations were normal. A mid-secretory phase progesterone level was 60 nmol l^{-1}. A semen analysis after 3 days' abstinence revealed a volume of 3 ml with azoospermia.

Q3: Which of the following would be reasonable options?
A: Donor insemination.
B: In vitro fertilization (IVF) with donor sperm.
C: Adoption.
D: None of the above.
E: Intrauterine insemination with sperm preparations.

The couple were devastated by this news and particularly so when the repeat semen analysis showed azoospermia.

Q4: How would you proceed?

The husband's follicle stimulating hormone (FSH) and luteinizing hormone (LH) levels were 3 and 4 IU l^{-1} respectively. A prolactin level was 160 mU l^{-1}. His karyotype was normal.

Q5: Which of the following would you advise?
A: Donor insemination.
B: IVF with donor sperm.
C: Testicular biopsy.
D: Adoption.
E: Intracytoplasmic sperm injection (ICSI).

After discussion, the decision to perform a testicular biopsy was taken. The biopsy showed that sperm production was taking place. A subsequent vasogram revealed bilateral congenital absence of the vas deferens.

Q6: What further options are available?

The couple did not feel in a position to afford specialized IVF, particularly when the likelihood of success was less than 70%. There was no guarantee that they would ever receive treatment within the National Health Service provision. After considerable discussion, they opted for donor insemination.

Q7: What investigations would you carry out before embarking on donor insemination?

Q8: What are the risks of donor insemination?

Q9: What are the chances of success with donor insemination?

Following three cycles of treatment, conception occurred and there was a successful outcome to the pregnancy.

COMMENTARY

The occurrence of subfertility is normally a shock to couples and it causes considerable anxiety. Such patients require careful consideration in an appropriate setting. The investigation and management of subfertility is time consuming and this needs to be made clear to the couple at the outset. They should be made aware of the possible causes. It is important that, as the involved physician, you are honest and do not give false or unrealistic hope to the couple (**Q1**).

Broadly, the investigations should address problems of ovulation, transport and male factors. In this case baseline hormonal levels should be measured in the woman including FSH, LH and thyroid function. Hyperprolactinaemia would be extremely unlikely in someone with regular cycles. The woman's rubella status should be ascertained. A mid-secretory phase progesterone level should be checked to confirm ovulation, and serial ultrasound scans may be undertaken to investigate follicular development and ovum release. There was no suggestion of a tubal problem in this case and you may choose not to investigate it at this stage, as both hysterosalpingography and laparoscopy are invasive procedures. Initial investigation of the male should be by semen analysis of a specimen produced at least 3 days after the most recent ejaculation (**Q2**).

Before acting on an abnormal semen analysis, you should always repeat this, particularly when the abnormality is azoospermia. Thus you should not advise donor insemination, IVF with donor sperm, or adoption after the first semen analysis (**Q3: true = D; false = A, B, C, E**).

Following the repeat confirmatory semen analysis, you should try to find out whether the problem is due to a failure of production, or of transport, from the testis. The karyotype should be checked, as should levels of FSH, LH and prolactin. Raised hormonal assays would suggest a failure of production. In this case, all the investigations were normal (**Q4**).

You should now recommend a testicular biopsy to confirm that spermatogenesis is occurring (**Q5: true = C; false = A, B, D, E (possibly)**). This was indeed the case, and the options for the male to father a child would now be by either IVF or investigation of the vas deferens to see whether or not there was a blockage that could be bypassed surgically. A vasogram was performed and it showed bilateral congenital absence of the vas deferens. Surgery was therefore not an option, and the couple was left with the alternatives of IVF, donor insemination or adoption. Interestingly, 50% of men with congenital absence of the vas deferens are carriers of the gene for cystic fibrosis, and, had the couple opted for IVF, they should have been counselled about screening. Had they wished to have IVF, you should have recommended intracytoplasmic sperm injection (ICSI) after surgical sperm recovery. Sperm is likely to be obtained in 100% of cases, and the clinical pregnancy rate is approximately 30% for each cycle (**Q6**).

Before embarking on donor insemination, it is important to assess the woman's tubal status. In the absence of any suggestion of a tubal problem, you should favour hysterosalpingography rather than laparoscopy. Ultrasonographic assessment of tubal potency is now possible, although not yet widely available (**Q7**).

The main risk of donor insemination is the transfer of serious viral infections from the donor, in particular hepatitis and human immunodeficiency virus (HIV). Frozen semen is now used so that testing can be carried out before insemination. Initial testing of the donor should be carried out before collection and freezing of semen. The donor should then be tested again for hepatitis and HIV 6 months later, before using the specimen. It is recommended that donors be screened for the cystic fibrosis gene. In addition, a careful personal and family history of psychiatric and genetic disorders should be taken (**Q8**).

With regard to success of donor insemination, Albrecht *et al* (1982) reported a pregnancy rate of 10–15% for each cycle (**Q9**).

REFERENCE

Albrecht BH, Cramer D, Schift I. Factors influencing the success of artificial insemination. *Fertil Steril* 1982; **37**: 792–797.

FACTS YOU SHOULD HAVE LEARNT . . .

- **The investigation and management of male subfertility**
- **The selection of donors and success rate of donor insemination.**

Index